# 1

# 'Will there be beds for me and all who seek?'

*Christina Rossetti*

---

*What is the problem?*

Christina Rossetti was not an early spokesman for the Patients' Association. Her interest was not in hospitals but inns. Her question, however, expresses the sentiments of patients and hospital staff alike and the answer is all too often 'No'. Year after year the daily pressure to find beds for emergency admissions causes stress to bed bureaux and hospitals. In some of our towns and cities, accident and emergency department staff have difficulty in arranging for the speedy admission of patients and are frequently at the centre of discordant negotiations between admission wards, 'on take' medical staff, senior nurses, administrators and bed bureaux staff. The pressures are not confined within hospital walls. General practitioners and the ambulance service find the difficulties of arranging admission frustrating and the patient himself may have to endure a long wait before getting into hospital. Some elderly patients are not admitted because it is claimed that their principal need for admission is based on social and domestic causes rather than purely clinical needs. The pressure on beds affects the planned admission policy of hospitals, leading to long delays for many waiting-list patients. A sudden influx of emergency admissions can lead to the cancellation of booked admission dates and the aggrieved patient may then complain to the hospital, the Health Service Commissioner, or his member of Parliament. The shortage of adequately staffed and supported hospital beds causes all sorts of reactions. One frustrated patient hijacked a hospital bed and then staged a 'sit-in' until she was operated upon. One consultant called a public meeting of his waiting-list patients in order to explain the problems he faced. Another consultant explained to the press, 'I have patients actually dying on my waiting list.' Both he and the health authority concerned agreed that 'the only solution is more money'. The problem of bed shortages seems long-lasting and acute. The solutions are only too often very short-term or depressingly distant – put up an extra bed or wait for a new hospital to be built.

There are just under half a million hospital beds in Great Britain today. In 1977, of the 459 000 staffed and available beds, 178 000 were allocated to psychiatry, 71 000 to geriatric medicine and units for the younger disabled and the remaining 210 000 were general hospital beds. The scope of this book is limited to these 210 000 so-called 'acute' hospital beds. Acute is something of a misnomer in that acute episodes of illness are regularly dealt with in psychiatric and geriatric hospitals and much of the care and treatment given in general hospitals is to those patients suffering from chronic illnesses. The so-called acute beds take a disproportionately large share of hospital revenue but they do receive over 90% of the more than six million annual admissions. They may not be 'acute' beds, but their availability appears to be an acute problem.

This book addresses itself to seeking solutions to the shortage of hospital beds on a time-scale that is considerably shorter than the wait for a new district general hospital. In so doing it has to challenge the view that 'the only solution is more money'. It is certainly one solution, it may be the best solution, but it is not the only solution. It is too easy for us to merely cry about the under-funding of the health service by successive governments. We must realise that more money for the National Health Service will almost certainly mean less for someone else. Approximately one person in every 25 employed in Great Britain works in the NHS, which takes over six per cent of the Gross National Product and in 1977 had an expenditure of over £7000 million. However good we are at securing value for money, surely there must be some scope for improvement – surely we can identify some wastage which can be saved and transferred to relieve our shortage of beds and save patients dying. Identifying certain kinds of savings in the NHS is easy: cut administrative costs, get rid of one level of authority, and reduce the number of porters on car parking duties! This type of saving should not be overlooked, but the money involved pales into insignificance against the cost of using hospital beds. Saving money is not just an option that we can choose to pick up or ignore. We must be realistic. More money for health is not going to be a solution in the immediate future, for the simple reason that both Government and Opposition policies are currently set against any significant increase in health service expenditure.

# HOSPITAL BEDS

# HOSPITAL BEDS

*A problem for diagnosis and management?*

*by*
## John Yates

*Research Associate,*
*Health Services Management Centre,*
*University of Birmingham*

William Heinemann Medical Books Ltd
London

First published 1982

© John Yates 1982

ISBN 0–433–37030–0

Photoset, printed and bound in Great Britain by
Redwood Burn Limited
Trowbridge, Wiltshire

# Contents

**To Ivy**

The study of inanimate statistics can be a soul-destroying activity, unless we remember that every hospital admission and day's stay has its own very personal story for each patient, his relatives and friends.

# Preface

The number of hospital beds and the way those beds are used are two interrelated issues which together form one of the platforms for a seemingly endless debate between doctors and administrators. For over twenty years much of the debate has concentrated on defining and providing the number of beds required, but recently, in the climate of financial stringency, there has been an increasing emphasis on how the existing bedstock is used.

This book is intended for doctors and all those who join with them in caring for patients in hospitals. In particular, it is aimed at two groups – the pessimistic who feel that no more can be achieved unless we increase our bedstock, and the optimistic who are prepared to attempt to make better use of existing resources. For the first group the book contains a challenge by demonstrating that we do not make the best use of our resources. For the second group it offers some guidance on methods of analysing the problems of bed use and reviews some of the ways of seeking improvement in that use. Unfortunately it demonstrates only too often how poor some of our analytical work has been and how unproven our solutions to problems appear to be. Health authority members and professional managers need to realise in what way their actions help or hinder clinicians in making good use of hospital beds. Whilst their support and occasional provocation is essential, I believe that it is the medical profession who must take the responsibility for ensuring that the best possible use is made of our hospitals. The results should be not merely beneficial to our budget but, more importantly, beneficial to our patients.

May 1982

John Michael Yates
Health Services Management Centre
University of Birmingham

# Acknowledgements

The gathering together of this material has been part of my study of the effectiveness and efficiency of clinical practice. The study has been funded by the Department of Health and Social Security and my work has been based at the Health Services Management Centre of the University of Birmingham.

The case studies in this book are taken from many hospitals in England. The interpretation of events is entirely personal, but the facts quoted are accurate and any action taken must be credited to the staff and authorities concerned, even though they are not named. All such case studies are presented in the text in small type.

My thanks go to Mr Eric Sweet for his excellent production of the diagrams and to many clinical, academic and administrative colleagues who have given me considerable help by reading drafts, discussing problems and making criticisms. At the risk of omitting important contributions I would like to thank Professor Gordon Cumming, Mr Mike Davidge, Mr Bob Dearden, Dr Alistair Geddes, Dr Dilip Karandikar, Mr David King, Mr Richard Shegog, Dr Peter Simpson, Mr Ron Spencer, Dr John Todd, Mrs Lorna Wainwright, Dr Don White and Dr Iden Wickings. My particular thanks go to Mr Brendan Devlin, Dr Alastair Mason, Mrs Lorna Vickerstaff and Dr Derek Williams who have not only helped to improve the book by their reading and research, but have also exhorted and encouraged me to complete it. Without Lorna's help and encouragement the manuscript would never have been completed.

Whilst the credit for any useful material must go to many colleagues, the responsibility for errors and omissions lies with myself.

# Foreword

*by Sir George Godber, formerly Chief Medical Officer, Department of Health and Social Security*

Modern health care requires a system of running review for two main reasons. The first is to ensure the greatest possible effectiveness of its procedures; the second to ensure that the best result is obtained from resources which are, and will remain, less than optimal. The NHS in particular needs continuous review because it must meet the needs of the whole population as best it can, and queueing is its only answer to overload. Responsibility for bed availability cannot be left to someone else. Over twenty years ago, when I was attempting to expound some analyses of hospital bed use to the Joint Consultants Committee, I was told by the then Chairman of the CCHMS that figures were a waste of time, it was sufficient that each consultant was satisfied that he had done his job effectively. My riposte to that was somewhat marred by my realisation that the table I had just circulated had a main column of figures in which the date had been added in to the total! It is not enough to have figures; they must also be accurate and at least intelligible enough for the average reader to notice an error like that.

The three Cogwheel Reports were all part of a gradual rapprochement between profession and department leading toward regular presentation of simple figures which Divisions could use in a running appraisal of their work. John Yates was one of those who tried to show how this could be done for Cogwheel III. This book goes much further, presenting clearly and briefly why we should look more closely at the way we use what we have, and suggests some simple forms of presentation that would help medical and other clinical staff to use what the administration can provide for them. The same kind of presentation should also help management. It is really time we stopped medical sniping at administration and looked for the beams in our own eyes. If John Yates succeeds in getting a few more clinicians to understand a Barber Johnson Diagram – and then to use it – the NHS will be quite a lot further on its way.

## Does the problem deserve attention?

Invariably, when you roll up your sleeves to tackle a problem, there is someone who criticises the way you tackle that problem and also suggests that it is not the real problem anyway. The doctors fighting the epidemic of cholera in London in 1854 could be criticised for their methods of treating individual patients and also for failing to address themselves to the source of the problem – the Broad Street pump. Even Dr John Snow's action in removing the pump handle so that water could not be obtained has been belittled by the suggestion that the epidemic was dying out anyway.

Those of us who choose to direct our attention to the problem of shortage of acute hospital beds must be aware of some of the criticisms that can quite reasonably be levelled against us. Firstly, we can be criticised for addressing the wrong problem. There are those who think we are obsessed with the hospital bed. In 1947 Richard Asher[5] said, 'It is always assumed that the first thing in any illness is to put the patient to bed. Hospital accommodation is always numbered in beds. Illness is measured by the length of time in bed. Doctors are assessed by their bedside manner. Bed is not ordered like a pill or a purge, but is assumed as the basis for all treatment.' Our continuing worries about shortages of beds need to be tempered by Asher's penetrating remarks. Do we really need the beds we claim to be short of, and do we make proper use of the beds that we have?

Even if society agrees that it is desirable for every person in pain to be admitted to a hospital bed if such a need is confirmed by a doctor, can we afford that ideal? The society of which patients and doctors are a part is not merely worried about expenditure. It wants to be assured that the care and treatment offered by hospitals is beneficial to individuals and the community. Concern is expressed about the harm that some medical technology is reputed to do, the doubtful effect of some treatment within hospital[32] and the doubtful value of hospital medicine in the face of lifestyle, human biology, environmental factors, and preventive and primary care medicine.[95 121] We are faced not merely with a problem of a shortage of hospital beds, but doubts about the efficacy, effectiveness and efficiency of hospital treatment. Both general usage and the dictionary definitions of these words blur three separate issues: (i) the ability of a course of action to make a change; (ii) the fact that a change is actually made; (iii) the best way of producing that change. In medicine, the word efficacy is used to denote that a drug has the ability to alter the natural history of a condition (usually for the better). The effectiveness of the drug, however, depends not only on the drug itself, but on the fact that it is correctly prescribed (the doctor advising the correct drug in the correct dosage) and that the patient complies with the regime. The efficiency of the treatment can then be seen as use of the least expensive of all suitable drugs in the minimum quantity necessary. In this book the three words are used with specific connotation: efficacy is the ability of something to make an alteration; effectiveness comments on the amount of success in making that alteration; efficiency aims at the least expensive way (not merely in terms of pounds) of producing the desired result. If we are uncertain about efficacy and effectiveness we cannot debate efficiency properly. As the National Health Service does not know sufficient about the efficacy and effectiveness of hospitals, it concerns itself with expenditure and pretends it is dealing with efficiency. The difficulties of measuring effectiveness and of linking information to enable satisfactory long-term follow-up of patients and their treatment take a back seat behind management systems designed to control expenditure. The situation we find ourselves in has been well described by Professor Calnan[24] who says, 'At the heart of the great British National Health Service there is a single inescapable flaw – inefficiency. To cover up for it we are all being asked to save money.' Examining a shortage of hospital beds may merely be an attempt to control expenditure rather than acquire knowledge of the efficacy and effectiveness of the hospital service. The solutions that this book seeks to find must be acknowledged as partial. Based on the assumption that a fair proportion of hospital activity is both efficacious and effective, it searches for ways of decreasing wasted resources and making better use of the beds we have today.

The second type of criticism is not so much that we are examining the wrong problem, but that we are examining the right problem in the wrong way. Concentrating on examining the hospital bed without a full study of all the other important resources such as staff, theatres, diagnostic facilities, etc., is obviously only doing part of the job. The criticism is fair, but it has to be recognised that the 'bed' often proves to be the dominant factor. When the demand for beds is high, hospital staff find great difficulty in resisting the use of those beds that are available. It is more common to see staffing and support services stretched to match bed provision than to find support services dictating the number of beds to be filled. As a very minimum, a study of beds should indicate whether it is the bed or some other factor which is a bottleneck in the efficient use of the whole hospital. Whether we like it or not, the number of hospital beds is a key factor in setting the tempo of a hospital's activity.

## Are there any solutions?

This book is written in the belief that there is a real problem and that it is worthy of attention. It accepts the evidence of staff and patient pressure groups that shortages occur with sufficient regularity to justify serious attention. However, it challenges the assumption that the only solution to the problem is to throw money at it – to provide more resources. It seeks other solutions and the approach adopted is in some ways similar to that used by clinicians in selecting diagnosis and treatment for individual patients. A consultant makes decisions about a patient's treatment which are based on information obtained from various sources. These include general practitioner letters, the consultant's own findings resulting from observation and examination, the results of pathological tests, the opinion of radiologist, and the patient's comments. Whilst some of this information may be inaccurate, incomplete, irrelevant, and even contradictory, diagnostic decisions are made, treatment is chosen and applied, and the patient usually recovers or improves. Within the medical process, diagnosis and treatment are often complex, treatments are sometimes of unproven value, and the placebo effect is encountered. The process of management which attempts to analyse and improve an organisation's performance is in many ways analogous to the diagnostic and treatment processes in medicine. I do not suggest that an organisation is like an individual patient, merely that the approach to problem-solving is very similar. The manager's task appears to lie predominantly in using doubtful information, dubious measures, uncertain diagnostic methods, and unproven treatment. Management is like the more uncertain, and perhaps more challenging, side of clinical practice. The framework of this book is based on this analogy.

# 2

# *Do we simply need more hospital beds?*

## SIGN, SYMPTOM OR DISEASE?

Disease in an organ or function of the body is recognised by the pattern of signs and symptoms. Even in a well-developed discipline like medicine, the understanding of and relationship between signs, symptoms, diseases and causes is incomplete, but in management the equivalent features of an organisation and its workings are far from clear.

This chapter attempts to distinguish between the surface problems and underlying dysfunctions of hospital beds. It suggests the examination of three related issues – the *amount*, the *use*, and the *spare capacity* of hospital beds.

---

### The Amount Of Bedstock

What are the factors that have determined the stock of beds in Great Britain or in any locality? In Fig. 1, bed stock is represented as a mass which has within it pressures to expand and yet at the same time its growth is being constrained and there are even pressures to contract. The size and shape of the mass is influenced by the internal (centrifugal) forces which try to increase the amount of bed stock. These forces include 'need' as determined by the medical profession and health services planners, and the influence of 'demand' as expressed by the population. When a patient feels unwell he decides whether or not to seek medical advice and thus makes a demand on the health service. The decision as to the patient's need for medical care is made by a doctor. Need commences as a professional judgement and as such may vary from doctor to doctor and from time to time. However, doctors

6

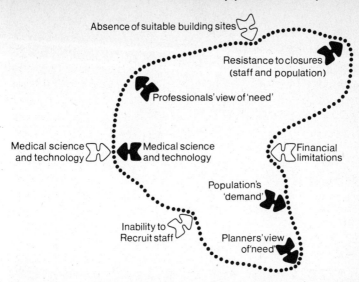

Absence of suitable building sites

Resistance to closures
(staff and population)

Professionals' view of 'need'

Medical science
and technology

Medical science
and technology

Financial
limitations

Population's
'demand'

Inability to
Recruit staff

Planners' view
of 'need'

Fig. 1   Some of the Forces that Influence the Amount of Bed Provision

who are placed in the position of determining the need for admission
are often influenced in making that decision by what is available in
resource terms. A review of the literature shows that the need for
hospital beds is a moving target. Assessments for the provision of acute
beds varied from 5·0 to 8·7 per 1000 population in 1945 to more recent
estimates of 2·0 to 2·5 per 1000 population. These rates are sometimes
called 'norms' and are used as a guideline in planning new hospitals.
The calculation of these norms has traditionally been based on surveys
of usage, refined by estimates of unmet demand, but these methods
have been shown to be highly influenced by the existing amount of provision at the time and place of the survey. To be cynical, norms are no
more than an historical look at an earlier age's provision, adjusted up
or down a little by today's prejudices. To be more specific, the DHSS's
latest view of provision for traumatic and orthopaedic surgery is a level
of 0·44 beds per 1000 population, whilst many orthopaedic surgeons
believe that the figure should be 0·55. The arithmetic mean of recent
years' provision is 0.44 but this hides a range from no provision at all in
one district to another which has one bed per thousand catchment
population. Even when agreement has been reached upon a desirable
ratio for a given region or area, there still appear to be difficulties

arising from the internal allocation within and between hospitals. A considerable volume of literature appears on the subject of need, but precise guidance which enables the measurement of prevalence of surpluses and deficiences is not easily available. Meredith *et al.* [104] provide a useful bibliography up to 1968, but more recent publications are available.[27 46]

These major issues of need and demand contain many elements. Advances in medical science can require additional provision of bed stock. At one time renal dialysis and hip replacement were not available, but newly-developed techniques have now made such treatments commonplace and thus increased the demand for additional resources, including hospital beds. The outward forces are not always entirely rational. Planners attempt to give under-provided areas a quantity of bed stock which will then enable a population to own what is considered a requisite stock, as determined by some norm. Whilst in theory such a force is based on the need determined by clinicians, the planning pressure can inadvertently result in a greater provision than can be used by the professionals. The imbalance is illustrated by newly-built district general hospitals, planned in an era when day-surgery, planned early discharge, improved anaesthetic techniques and new drugs were not anticipated, and the result is over-provision.[45] Another outward force is that of civic fear and pride, which requires every hamlet, village, town and district of a city to press for its own hospital, regardless of need or the practicalities of staffing. The outward forces not only seek to expand provision, but also resist contraction. Staff, their unions, and the community frequently resist closures which are proposed, even if such closure is supported on clinical, financial or operational grounds. Finally, expansion is caused by the sort of inappropriate bed use which will be described later in this chapter.

Figure 1 also shows forces which oppose the expansion of bed provision and even seek to reduce provision. One of the more forceful pressures is that of financial constraint. Limitations on public expenditure can deter expansion and also call for a reduction in provision. Other factors include the inability to recruit staff and the difficulties of obtaining suitably placed building sites. Some of these inward pressures come from the same sources that provide pressures for expansion. Developments in medical science not only call for additional resources but, at the same time, reduce requirements for bed provision. In psychiatry, the use of psychotropic drugs has greatly changed patterns of care, allowing very many patients who were formerly institutionalised to be kept (permanently under supervision) in the community.

Similarly, in other specialities, the development of specific pharmacological agents (streptomycin for tuberculosis; metronidazole in the management of appendicectomy; cimetidine for peptic ulceration) has influenced to varying degrees the admission rates and length of stay of medical and surgical patients, and has consequently had an effect upon the bed provision required. It is not only the development of new drugs that reduces the amount of bed provision. New operative techniques and investigatory procedures can have similar effects, and practising clinicians are not slow to see the implications of such developments. The introduction of circular stapling devices for making intestinal and similar anastomoses has enabled surgeons to carry out operations which were undreamed of years ago. Thus in general surgery the requirements for hospital beds for the treatment of a common condition, rectal cancer, is likely to diminish. Although this equipment is expensive, it is very cost-effective in use and should greatly reduce the amount of work in the hospital and in the community nursing services. For instance, it was reported by R. J. Heald[68] that in one year, instead of carrying out 27 abdominoperineal resections of the rectum with the consequent long postoperative stay in hospital, he had treated all but seven of his rectal cancers using a circular stapling device, and had been able to get the majority of his patients home within a few days. This represents a very considerable saving in hospital beds.

These centrifugal and centripetal forces are difficult to quantify and classify. They appear to vary in intensity from place to place and over time. It is important to note that some of these forces not only work in both directions, but sometimes do so at the same time. Political pressures, for instance, can call for more provision for the dying and the reduction of the waiting list, yet also require the reduction of public expenditure, including that on health. The other interesting feature is that adjustments to the amount of provision take place over a long time-scale. An organisation as large as our health service needs time to react to changing situations. This is most noticeable in bed deficiency circumstances when the timelag between perceiving the existence of a deficiency and correcting that deficiency involves the planning, building, and commissioning of a new hospital. This activity is seldom done in less than five years, and usually takes ten. Changes in bed stock are not only upward. In some localities, specialties are faced with a decrease, and some specialties move through a long period of reduction in bed stock. In tuberculosis, for example, falling bed numbers are due to the decreasing incidence of tuberculosis and the changes in admission and length of stay patterns.

CASE STUDY
Fig. 2 shows the bed availability and occupancy of three hospitals over a period of 16 years. The average emptiness for the whole period is 27% and the monthly variation was from 7% to 50% of beds empty. The three hospitals took patients with chest diseases and tuberculosis. In each hospital, wards were designated for tuberculosis and nontuberculous patients and wards were also separately allocated to males, females and children. The clinicians responsible for the clinical care of the patients reviewed the use of resources on a six-monthly basis for the whole of the period, and recommended adjustments in bed provision accordingly. Amongst the factors that they had to take into account were the impracticability of reducing bed complements in blocks of less than a ward at a time; the need to decorate and maintain premises; the transferring of wards to specialties in such a way that nursing and other staff were not made redundant; and the need to have beds always available for male, female and child admissions for chest disease and tuberculosis patients in the event of influenza epidemics. Changes in the incidence of tuberculosis caused by a growing immigrant community had also to be considered.

The case study and the previous discussion illustrate that the amount of bed stock is influenced by the amount of spare capacity required and also by the way in which the occupied beds are used. Figure 3 attempts to illustrate the relationship between these three issues. For example, when the amount of bed provision is inadequate this might cause undue pressure on spare capacity, but at the same time it encourages the efficient use of beds and minimises inappropriate use. These two issues, spare capacity and inappropriate use, require separate examination.

## The Amount Of Reserve Capacity Required

The driver of a number 96 bus once said, 'If there are five empty seats and I say the bus is full, the bus is full.' I suspect that he was married to a ward sister!

Hospitals need some empty beds to function properly, but the problem is to decide how many. Empty beds are frequently included in discussions about the amount of provision and, whilst obviously related, the subject really deserves separate consideration. Spare capacity is required to deal with the unpredictability of admission rates, length of stay, and the mixture of sex and condition of patients. No hospital can be fully staffed and equipped to cope with all the fluctuations that might be encountered without having a high level of unused beds and underemployed staff. Even if possible fluctuations

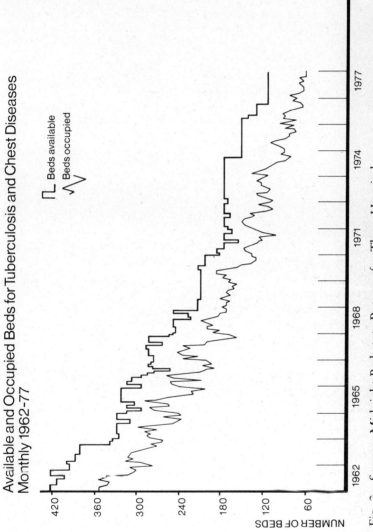

Available and Occupied Beds for Tuberculosis and Chest Diseases
Monthly 1962-77

⌐⌐ Beds available

〜 Beds occupied

NUMBER OF BEDS

420
360
300
240
180
120
60

1962  1965  1968  1971  1974  1977

Fig. 2    Source: Midnight Bed-state Returns for Three Hospitals.

## The Relationship between Amount, Spare Capacity, and Use of Hospital Beds

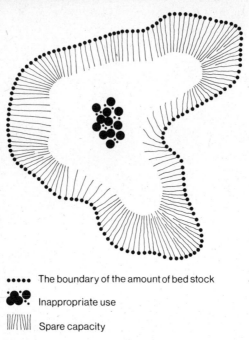

••••• The boundary of the amount of bed stock

Inappropriate use

Spare capacity

Fig. 3

caused by major accidents and epidemics are discounted, there is still a wide band of possible admission rates and bed occupancy.

Emergency admissions are generally distributed in a random fashion. When grouped into large numbers it is possible to assess what size of facility, including spare capacity, is required to cope with demand, but the number of emergency admissions for one day or one specialty in one hospital cannot be predicted with any certainty. This justifies having a unit large enough to cope with the higher end of the fluctuating demand if no alternative facility is available. Additionally, it is generally accepted that the constant use of beds is not only unobtainable but is undesirable. It is necessary to allow sufficient time to change bedding, clean and maintain the bedstead and the immediate environment, and also give ward staff some respite. When an allowance is made for a gap (turnover interval) between one discharge and the next admission, it must be recognised that the higher the number of patients admitted the lower the attainable bed occupancy. The amount of spare capacity can be enlarged or distorted by the need to make separate provision for male, female and child admissions, the provision of allocations for individual specialty or consultant use and the need to cater for seasonal trends, such as the higher use of medical wards for emergencies during winter. Spare capacity is related to many variables and in consequence few are prepared to suggest general standards which specify the amount required, but attempts to provide a baseline of acceptable or required bed emptiness appear in the work of a number of authors.[113][72] These papers include the examination of the unpredictability of demand for beds and discuss the use of the Poisson distribution and other techniques in attempting to predict demand and minimise the number of empty beds. This type of work can give some indication of a figure above which bed surplus can be assumed, but all the work illustrates the many factors involved in calculating the amount of slack required and any figures provided relate to specific wards and specialties rather than whole hospitals or regional and national standards.

Returning to Fig. 3, it is possible to visualise pressures which expand and compress the area of spare capacity. Forces to expand include the expectation of both staff and patients that minimal work should be undertaken at weekends, bank holidays, and certain other increasing holiday periods, and thus higher emptiness occurs at these times. Further pressure is caused by the inability to balance the supply, standard, and timing of staffing and support services, resulting in an enlargement of the amount of spare capacity. To attain maximum use of all departments is difficult and full use of one department can mean under-use of another. The amount of spare capacity can also be expanded by industrial action, both within and outside the hospital. Compression is caused by such pressures as over-optimistic cold admission policies, failure to make adequate allowance for the variations in normal emergency admissions, and the occurrence of major accidents or epidemics. The amount of spare capacity can be heavily influenced by the amount of provision; too much provision, for example, usually results in too much spare capacity.

## The Way In Which Beds Are Used

'Logan's third law of thermodynamics is reputed to be that a hospital bed must be kept warm'. The dangers of bed use illustrated by Asher,[5] and the cost of providing beds, place upon us the need to ensure that bed use is appropriate. Should the patient be admitted at all? How long should the patient stay? In what type of accommodation should the patient be? Variations in practice are evident in all three areas but the question of whether such variations indicate some inappropriate use is difficult to ascertain. Three 'diseases' are, however, identifiable; unnecessary admission, unnecessary stay, and incorrect location. These may at first sight appear to be matters of a solely clinical nature, but organisational and environmental factors can be seen to influence the admission, stay and location of patients. As an example consider the following case-study:

CASE STUDY

The weekly emergency admissions in general medicine for a large city are shown in Fig. 4 for the first six months of 1973, 1974 and 1975. The normal pattern of emergency medical admissions (unless an unusual epidemic occurs) is for a general decrease in admissions over the six-month period. The marked decline during March 1973 is unusual for two reasons. Firstly, it is rare for emergency admissions to drop below 300 per week during the winter months and, secondly, it is uncommon to see a change of such magnitude in only one week (89 less cases in week ending March 4th than February 25th). The period coincides with the negotiations between ancillary staffs and the DHSS and the subsequent two-week strike. It had been claimed that the strike would not affect emergencies. During the period there was no evidence of a change in the mortality rate for the city, although other effects, such as increased morbidity because of delayed admission, were not quantified.

The case-study raises the issue of the extent to which patients, general practitioners and the hospital doctors altered their criteria about the need for emergency admission immediately before and during the strike. If the same criteria were always applied then the need for hospital beds would be considerably reduced! Doctors frequently disagree openly about the need for admission, the appropriate length of stay, and the correct location for their patients. The medical literature abounds with debate about the necessity of admission for medical investigations and for operative surgery. Differences in practice are easily observed and some are very easily explained. Different admission rates from different neighbourhoods of the same city are understandable if social conditions and standards of primary care facilities are demonstrably different. On the other hand, some of the longer periods of stay and higher admission rates are difficult to understand, particularly in areas where there are observed shortages of beds. Any search for the

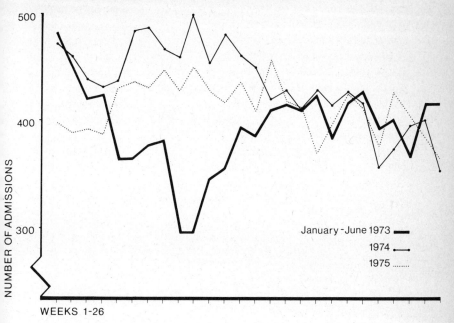

Fig. 4    Source: Daily records of the City's Bed Bureau.

prevalence of inappropriate admission, length of stay, and location of patients will invariably lead to small local studies which cannot easily be projected to assess national levels.

**Unnecessary admissions**

Todd[137] gives examples of unnecessary admissions for investigation, and many others suggest day-case surgery instead of hospital admission, e.g. Ruckley.[127] Gainsborough[56] in reviewing papers on the subject of unnecessary admission, found, at one extreme, estimates of 25% of male and 40% of female patients having no diagnostic or therapeutic need for admission, with a figure as low as 4% at the other extreme. In addition to differences in clinical practice, the admission decisions are influenced by other factors such as the patient's views, the patient's home circumstances, the availability of resources, and the policies of the hospital to which the patient is admitted. West and Carey[142] in examining variations of between 0·64 and 2·04 per 1000 population in admission rates for appendicitis conclude that 'admission rates vary mainly because of differing admission policies. Admission is not wholly governed by the sudden onset of abdominal pain; other factors include, the threshold of consultation of each patient, the referral habits of general practitioners, the availability of hospital beds and the degree to which doctors and patients expect admission.' Mawson and Stroud[103] note the parental pressure for childrens' tonsil and adenoid operations, Logan *et al.*[88] suggest that higher levels of hospital provision encourage higher levels of admission rates, and Wynne and Hull[148] point out that 20% of paediatric admissions are primarily for social reasons. This latter case, however, illustrates the difficulties of making a judgement about appropriate admission. Admissions may be clinically and therapeutically unnecessary and yet society may choose, and possibly should choose, to use its hospital beds to admit such patients.

## Unnecessary length of stay

Apart from the patient's presenting characteristics such as age, disease and condition, three other groups of factors appear to influence length of stay. These are the clinical policies of the medical staff, the organisational and administrative habits of the doctors and hospitals, and the extra-hospital influences of social environment and availability of paramedical support services to which the patient is to be discharged. Identifying and separating these factors can be difficult. Variations in clinical practice were noted by Gilkes and Handa[60] in a review of clinical policies of pre- and postoperative cases in ophthalmology. Other examples are published, e.g. Harpur[66] examining early discharge of uncomplicated acute myocardial infarction cases, and Heasman[69] studying tonsillectomy, adenoidectomy and inguinal hernias. Organisational and administrative influences include strict adherence to ward round discharge days, failure to balance admission and operating days, and lack of pressure on hospitals. Examples of this type of factor are published by Hunter.[77] Reasons for inappropriate stay classified under the heading 'social environment' are usually related to inadequate home conditions, particularly for elderly patients with no family assistance and no alternative appropriate accommodation in geriatric beds or social service hostels, e.g. Rubin and Davies,[126] Strang *et al.*,[135] Murphy.[111]

## Incorrect location

Beds which have staffing support and equipment specifically designed for one purpose can be inappropriately occupied by patients not requiring that level of care. One national study by Meredith *et al.*[104] suggests that up to 36% of district general hospital beds were occupied by patients who could have been in more suitable alternative accommodation. Loudon[90] states that, whilst 1% of general medical admissions appeared inappropriate, 17% of patients reviewed during his study were not in the right type of accommodation. Incorrect location of patients appears to be a more common occurrence than unnecessary admission.

Returning again to Fig. 3, the desire of both medicine and management to avoid inappropriate bed use is clearly subject to many pressures. Explanations for real or apparent inappropriate use include the quite rational action of a clinician who has some doubt about diagnosis or the severity of the condition and chooses to allow time for observation. Whilst retrospective analysis of his action might show that the period of observation was unnecessary, few would suggest that it would not be rational to allow some margin of apparently inappropriate use. Lack of social service provision, lack of home nursing cover, failure to distribute knowledge about well-established clinical practice, failures to schedule admission, discharge, and investigation procedures, and failing to have admission screening by a senior clinician are all factors which cause inappropriate use of beds. Some staff are known to encourage longer stay for some patients in order to keep beds full. Motivation for this type of action includes defending the ward from having to take emergency cases, saving the bed for planned admissions, and even using fully-occupied wards as a bargaining tactic when seeking more resources.

## Distinct But Not separate?

The amount, spare capacity and use of hospital beds each have their own dysfunctions or 'diseases'. The three elements are, however, almost inseparable and each affects the others. Identifying precisely what problems exist in a hospital is not always easy. Look for example at the following case studies.

CASE STUDY 1
An eighteen-year-old girl who has just taken an overdose of tablets arrives at an accident and emergency department at 10.00 p.m. The medical registrar decides that she needs to be admitted but all the female

medical wards are full. If he suggests an extra bed is erected on one of the wards he will incur the wrath of the nursing staff, who will point out that nurses who are already over-stretched cannot be expected to cope with an additional work-load. None of the empty male beds in the main male medical wards can be used and the few single cubicles on the male medical wards are already occupied by seriously ill patients. He has no scope for transferring patients within his own specialty. The surgical registrar has only two vacant 'female' beds. He is unwilling to assist the medical registrar and points out that there are already ten medical cases occupying beds in the ninety allocated surgical beds and he has to keep the two empty 'female' beds for emergency surgical admissions. He anticipates that the number of surgical emergencies during the night will be greater than the beds he has available. The medical registrar's enquiries of other specialties reveal a similar picture. The only glimmer of hope comes from the infectious diseases unit. The unit is prepared to co-operate by loaning a few beds, but points out that the available beds are in isolation cubicles which are not equipped or staffed for the type of medical emergency proposed. Thoughts of transferring the girl to another hospital are impracticable – they claim to be just as busy and, even if beds were available, the process of transferring a fairly ill patient is seen as inadvisable. The girl is eventually admitted to an infectious diseases ward and two days later she is sufficiently recovered to be discharged.

CASE STUDY 2
One hospital sends admission notices to its planned admission cases requesting that the patient telephones the hospital between 11.20 a.m. and 12.00 noon to check that a bed is available. If a bed is available the patient is requested to attend by 1.00 p.m. The admission notice is usually received by patients one or two days before admission, regardless of the number of months or years the patient has been waiting for an operation. The letter explains that the reason for this tight schedule is the high pressure on hospital beds. The hospital in question has a turnover interval of seven days! (i.e. on average there is a seven-day gap between one patient's day of discharge and the next patient's admission). In the same city all other acute hospitals and all units of the same specialty consider themselves under pressure and yet all have shorter turnover intervals. A throughput of 30 cases per bed per year in the hospital concerned compares with similar units of 50–70 cases per bed per year.

Even with more information than is presented, it is difficult to make judgements about the appropriateness of the allocation and use of beds. The first case involved the eighteen-year-old girl. The staff of the hospital concerned were adamant in their feeling that they had too few beds. The bed occupancy in general medicine, general surgery and traumatic and orthopaedic surgery was consistently over 90%. The average gap between one discharge and the next admission was always less than a day. Many of us would have sympathy for the frustrations felt by the staff concerned, but the issue is not clear-cut. Similar hospitals elsewhere in the country with comparable patient loads had a length of stay in general medicine which was four days shorter than the hospital in the case study. In the surgical specialties little use was made of day unit facilities. To some extent it could be argued that the hospital staff were providing a rod for their own back by failing to use short-stay and day-case practice. In the second case study the hospital appeared to be a little behind the times. Its administration did not seem to arrange patient admissions satisfactorily and throughput appeared to be somewhat out of step with other similar units. A seven-day gap between one discharge and the next admission for an acute hospital clearly seems to indicate too many beds. But perhaps there were reasons, such as trouble with staffing levels and operating theatre provision and an unusual case-mix. Perhaps they were working efficiently but merely failed to record the statistics correctly!

The pioneers of medicine were confronted with the difficulties of understanding and defining symptoms, diseases, and causes. Even today the separation of these entities is not always completely clear. Dysmenorrhoea and schizophrenia for example, appear as diseases in the International Classification of Diseases but are regarded by many only as symptoms. In management, difficulties arise through our lack of precision in the use of certain terms. We need to make a clear distinction between the problems themselves and the manifestations and causes of those problems.

When the amount of bed provision is incorrectly established a number of 'signs and symptoms' or characteristics can occur. In the same way that one symptom is unlikely to indicate precisely a particular disease, so the existence of one characteristic alone cannot identify a dysfunction in the running of hospitals. The amount of bed provision can be too large or too small. When it is too small, some of the characteristics that can occur include:

## 1. Unnecessary time and effort spent in securing admission
In most cities this problem occurs within and between hospitals. In major district general hospitals it is not uncommon for medical, nursing or administrative staff to make over a dozen telephone calls to secure an admission. Wards are contacted to ascertain the latest bed state position and inter-ward transfers have to be arranged. Admiss-

ions are sometimes kept waiting on trolleys in the accident and emergency department. Relatives complain, staff tempers rise and morale falls. Patients are even kept in the accident and emergency departments until a patient can be discharged. Transfers between hospitals are not uncommon and it is not unknown for an ambulance to call at several hospitals before securing an admission.

## 2. 'Bed borrowing'

Bed borrowing or lodging out within hospitals, and the admission of patients to hospitals further away from their home than is normal, are two further symptoms of bed deficiency. Borrowing beds from other wards or specialties can cause difficulties for nurses, doctors and patients. The nurses on an infectious diseases ward, whilst competent to nurse an overdose admission, are working in an environment which is physically designed and specially equipped for infectious diseases. The nurses' interest often lies within a particular discipline and specialties frequently require different skills and varying staffing levels. Bed borrowing requires the doctor to visit more wards and thus reduces the time he has available and also increases the time it takes to call him to a patient. Bed borrowing can cause patient care to be less than optimal. An increasing incidence of transfers can mean a loss of continuity of nursing care and sometimes leads to problems with loss of patients' property. A sudden admission to the wrong ward may also affect a patient who was booked as a waiting list admission.

## 3. Extra beds

An alternative to bed borrowing is the erection of extra beds on a ward. Whilst there are no figures to support the contention that this method is less frequently used than hitherto, it is certainly true that newer ward designs do not facilitate the cramming of beds that was possible in the 'Nightingale' design wards. Extra beds are nevertheless a regular feature in some hospitals. Additional nurse staffing seldom occurs in parallel and thus additional pressure is placed on existing staff. General medical unit complements of 100 beds have been known to be filled with up to 120 patients through the erection of extra beds.

## 4. Early discharge

High pressure on hospital beds can encourage clinical staff to examine the patients on the ward carefully to see which patient is most able to go home in order to make space for an incoming admission. Whilst this can be a useful incentive to make the best use of beds, it does sometimes lead to the discharge of patients earlier than is clinically or socially desirable. On occasions, clinical staff are faced with resource constraints affecting the decision of whether a patient must die at home or in hospital.

## 5. High throughput
A high throughput can lead to a drop in standards of care. Situations where day-cases occupy the beds of ambulant in-patients, or a bedstead has been occupied by more than two patients in one day, are far from ideal.

## 6. Creation, maintenance or growth of a waiting list
Pressure on beds results in priority being given to the urgent cases at the expense of the less urgent. If the less urgent cases do not have to be admitted, they are placed on a waiting list for planned admission. Continuing pressure on beds from urgent cases can block beds for planned admissions and the waiting lists grow and waiting time lengthens. Waiting lists can be created for other reasons such as theatre or staff shortages, and it should not be assumed that they exist only because of a shortage of beds.

When the amount of bed provision is too large, few obvious characteristics occur and none of these is solely associated with a surplus. Three events which can occur simultaneously are: low staff morale because of inactivity; comparatively long duration of patient stay in relation to normal patterns for similar diagnostic groups; and slack thinking in terms of diagnostic work-up of patients.  Perhaps the most usual feature is that of a complete absence, over a long period, of all the characteristics associated with bed deficiency. To distinguish between an apparent numerical surplus and an actual usable surplus is difficult. Case Study 1 illustrated that an empty bed is not necessarily a suitable bed. It is also necessary to recognise that, after a while, nurse staffing will be adjusted to take account of a unit or hospital's consistent over-provision. Staff are transferred to other units and shorter working hours are absorbed without the need to claim additional revenue, then, when pressure is suddenly exerted in the form of additional admissions or longer length of stay, the unit is unable to work at its presumed full capacity.

Having examined the 'signs and symptoms' associated with dysfunction in the amount of bed provision, it would be apposite to list the features of excess and insufficient spare capacity and of inappropriate use of beds. In fact, however, inappropriate bed use, whether judged by admissions or length of stay, is accompanied by few specific characteristics, and whilst certain features commonly occur, they are by no means a sure sign that bed use is inappropriate. Excessive regularity of discharge patterns might suggest that discharge is determined by the date of the ward round rather than by need, but operating theatre schedules and planned early discharge schemes might cause incorrect conclusions to be drawn. Two further characteristics include the existence of long gaps between admission and operation or diagnostic investigation and comparatively long length of stay, low through-put and high admission rates for the case mix. The characteristics which accompany inappropriate location can include shortage of capacity, e.g. surgical beds blocked by geriatric cases, but yet again inappropriate use is not necessarily the causative factor. Inappropriate use of beds can in theory be eliminated, but probably only at the risk of some patients being discharged too early and others not being admitted – thus creating problems of inappropriate discharge and inappropriate exclusion!

In summary, the apparently simple problem of providing a sufficient quantity of hospital beds is complicated by many forces such as advances in medical technology and science, changes in public attitude and financial restrictions. It is also complicated by the fact that the amount of bed stock is one of three interrelated factors. The separate examination of these three factors of the amount, spare capacity and use of hospital beds is in itself difficult when:

1. The factors are so closely interrelated.
2. Indications of failure (signs and symptoms) are not specific.
3. Precise diagnostic tools are not readily available.
4. We are unclear about true values of what is or is not appropriate.

# 3

# *What information is available?*

## BASIC MEASUREMENTS AND SPECIAL INVESTIGATION.

Signs and symptoms alone are not always enough to make or confirm a diagnosis. Further aids in the diagnostic process include many types of measurement, for example, the patient's temperature, blood pressure, haemoglobin level and ESR. Some measurements are undertaken continuously and others are taken on one or two specific occasions. The measurement of an organisation's activity does not have the precision of some of medicine's aids, but in the same way uses both routinely collected information and *ad hoc* studies.

This chapter describes the three main sources of routinely collected information and comments on the intended use, actual use and criticisms of each system.

---

Few people find hospital statistics exciting. Most doctors and administrators dismiss them as inaccurate and in any case would not feel that mere figures could help examine a problem such as a shortage of beds. In the circumstances described in Chapter 1 it might be thought that the hijacker was either skilled or fortunate to find an empty bed. According to hospital statistics, that was not necessarily so; it was one of over 60 000 acute beds which can be empty on any day in Great Britain. The recorded number of empty, yet staffed, available beds has grown both in proportion and in real terms for many years. The statistical picture of idle capacity does not match our feelings of intense pressure, so should we dismiss the figures as inaccurate and misleading? Are the figures wrong, can they be justified, or can we make better use of our hospital beds?

When examining the acute hospital statistics it is only too easy to find errors. There are, for example, failures to record ward closures for decoration or to note reductions in bed complement because of staffing shortages. Both of these give a false picture of the number of beds available for use. Even when staffed available beds are correctly counted, there can be no guarantee that other resources, such as theatre capacity or diagnostic facilities can match the available beds. In addition to errors of fact, there are also problems of interpretation. Does the hospital bed in any way represent the work-load and pressures of a hospital? In recent years there have been enormous changes in methods of investigation and treatment, which have taken much care and cure away from the bed to out-patient departments, day-care units and the patient's home.

Despite these misgivings, an examination of the crude national figures does confirm some of our feelings. Hospital staff know that they have seen more patients than before, and Table 1 confirms that view. In addition to the known growth in day-case investigation and surgery, there was a 20% increase in the number of discharges and deaths between 1964 and 1979. Table 1 shows that NHS staff are justifiably indignant to find their performance measured by the size of the waiting list rather than by their productivity. Increasing patient numbers have been achieved against a decrease in the number of beds available. The annual increase in discharges and deaths was interrupted on only two occasions – in 1973 and 1975. These exceptions come as no surprise to NHS staff, who are aware that industrial action on a scale not previously seen occurred in those two years. Whether the industrial action caused the decrease in throughput is perhaps open to some debate, but many staff see a strong, if not direct, relationship.

Whilst this examination of the figures shows some harmony with the feelings of NHS staff, these same figures demonstrate that on average, between 51 000 and 64 000 beds are empty daily! Figure 5 shows that a steady decrease in bed stock from 1964 to 1976 was converging with a steady increase in the number of empty beds. Only since 1977 has the number of empty beds started to slowly decline in parallel with the decreasing bed stock. The consistent growth in spare capacity up to 1976, paralleled by a growth in throughput (Fig. 6) might at first appear a paradox, but to some extent they are complementary rather than conflicting issues. Increasingly, throughput may well require some proportionate growth in spare capacity. If a constant gap is allowed after each discharge, then the more discharges the larger the amount of spare capacity required. Increased throughput could be a

*Table 1*

'Acute' hospital beds and patients – Great Britain 1964–1979

| 1 year | 2 available beds (thousands) | 3 occupied beds (thousands) | 4 discharges and deaths (thousands) | 5 average length of patient stay (days) | 6 waiting list numbers (thousands) |
|---|---|---|---|---|---|
| 1964 | 230 | 178 | 4978 | 13.1 | 530 |
| 1965 | 230 | 178 | 5079 | 12.8 | 549 |
| 1966 | 229 | 176 | 5149 | 12.5 | 572 |
| 1967 | 229 | 174 | 5276 | 12.0 | 572 |
| 1968 | 229 | 172 | 5414 | 11.6 | 570 |
| 1969 | 227 | 170 | 5554 | 11.2 | 595 |
| 1970 | 224 | 166 | 5599 | 10.8 | 588 |
| 1971 | 225 | 165 | 5774 | 10.4 | 559 |
| 1972 | 223 | 163 | 5823 | 10.2 | 547 |
| 1973 | 220 | 157 | 5704 | 10.0 | 591 |
| 1974 | 219 | 157 | 5764 | 9.9 | 596 |
| 1975 | 215 | 151 | 5525 | 10.0 | 667 |
| 1976 | 214 | 150 | 5797 | 9.5 | 686 |
| 1977 | 210 | 149 | 5889 | 9.2 | 679 |
| 1978 | 207 | 150 | 5966 | 9.2 | 768 |
| 1979 | 204 | 147 | 5981 | 9.2 | 784 |

Source: 1964–76 from Health and Personal Social Services Statistics for England (summary tables for Great Britain published 1973 and 1977); 1977–9 are unpublished figures obtained from the DHSS and the Scottish Health Services Common Services Agency.

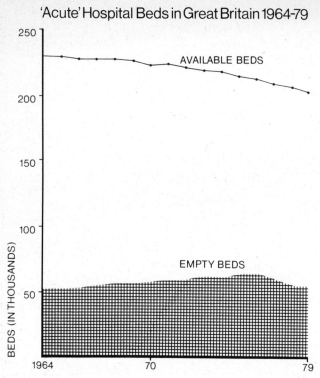

Fig. 5   Source: Table 1

powerful explanation for the increasing number of empty beds. In more recent years, the effects of industrial action by staff may well have influenced throughput but, despite industrial action, throughput continues to rise and, although spare capacity is no longer increasing, we are still left with over 28% of our acute hospital beds empty.

A figure of 57 000 empty beds is not easily reconciled with the long waiting lists and the difficulties in containing emergency admissions discussed in Chapter 1. Our cursory glance at national hospital statistics has on the one hand confirmed some of our feelings whilst, on the other hand, providing a nagging doubt about the number and proportion of empty available beds. Examining local statistics only serves to increase curiosity. The variations between specialties and between districts and hospitals are often so large that it is sometimes difficult to argue for more beds until we have justified the use or non-use of those we have. Whilst 28% of all acute beds in 1977 were empty, some specialties like traumatic and orthopaedic surgery were making much

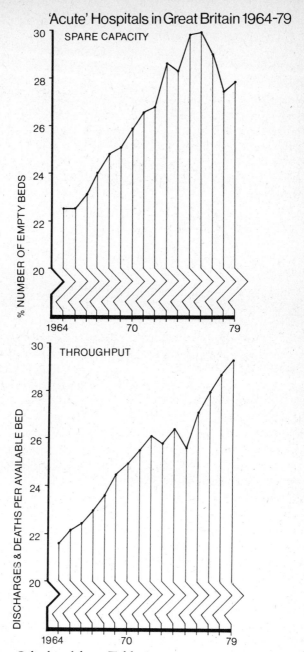

Fig. 6   Source: Calculated from Table 1

heavier use of beds, with only 18% of their stock empty – yet district by district the range of empty beds ranged from 0–60% in that specialty.

Before making any further study of such statistics we need to know more about their accuracy, value, and even their availability. Too often both doctors and administrators avoid the effort required to understand and correct the available information. It is easy to make sweeping criticisms of a subject in order to hide ignorance and justify unwillingness to spend time on improving the imperfect. The remainder of this chapter attempts to provide doctors with a ten-minute introduction to the statistics about hospital beds, and provides a large number of references for anyone who wishes to pursue the subject in more depth.

## Routinely Collected Information

The three principal sources of information about hospital beds are the *Midnight Bed State Returns* (summarised to complete Annual Hospital Returns – Form SH3), the *Hospital In-Patient Enquiry* (HIPE) and *Hospital Activity Analysis* (HAA).

**Midnight bed state returns and annual hospital returns – Form SH3**
Since 1948, hospitals in England and Wales have been asked to provide statistics annually on Form SH3. Each year, hospitals receive guidance from the DHSS on the completion of returns (e.g. DHSS[42]) and this guidance has ensured a basic similarity both in information systems and the data collected, although many variations exist between hospitals.

Typically each hospital collects daily information (between midnight and 9.00 a.m.) about bed availability, bed occupancy and admissions and discharges for each ward and specialty. At a local level, information can be made available on a daily, monthly, quarterly or annual basis, but on a national scale the information is collected annually. Whilst some of the Form SH3 content has changed over the years, it remains the only source of information about hospital bed use which has been continually and comparably available for all National Health Service hospitals. It has consistently recorded basic measurements of provision and utilisation of services, e.g. available and occupied beds, discharges and deaths, waiting list numbers, outpatient attendances and basic information about departments such as radiology and pathology. Annual reports containing this information are published for the whole of Great Britain (e.g. DHSS[43]).

The purpose of collecting this information is to obtain a national picture to aid the planning of future services and also to provide information locally about the use of resources. The following criticisms have been made of the system:

1. It is not possible to make analyses based on diagnosis, age, sex, residential area or consultant in charge of the patients. For example, there is no way of separating deaths in hospital from discharges (except at a local level) and it is not possible to identify the number of children who were admitted to surgical wards.

2. The importance of accuracy is not always recognised by the staff who collect the information and any system which yields annual figures by adding and carrying forward daily counts from individual wards to the DHSS runs the risk of haphazard arithmetic. For some years, the remuneration of administrators and other hospital staff was governed by the bed allocation figure and 'paper' figures were not uncommon.

3. The information is related to events rather than to individuals. There is no way of determining the number of readmissions or of identifying an individual patient from SH3 information.

4. There are classification anomalies and there has in the past been slowness in correcting such anomalies when recognised. For example, apparent differences in length-of-stay patterns between hospitals can be explained by the presence or absence of long-stay or preconvalescent discharge facilities. Morris *et al.*[110] stated, 'Among the most irrational of the long-standing anomalies which have been rectified recently were the instructions regarding calculation of the average bed availability, which did not allow for temporary "borrowing" of beds between specialties, leading to the production of meaningless figures for such derived indices as the bed turnover rate and turnover interval.'

Despite these and other criticisms the Midnight Returns and SH3 Forms remain the most up-to-date information base for hospital management at both operational and planning levels. At hospital level, the emergency admission arrangements usually involve the manipulation and supplementing of Midnight Return data.[30 61 134] Within and between hospitals the review of bed allocation and bed use frequently relies on SH3 information.[82 110 131 143]

**Hospital In-Patient Enquiry (HIPE)**

In 1949, in-patient summaries for a national morbidity enquiry were first collected in a small number of hospitals. Information was originally collected on all discharges, but from 1953 the enquiry was limited to a 10% sample. It was 1958 before full coverage of all non–psychiatric hospitals was achieved. The information collected relates to the patient himself, the administrative arrangements at the hospital for the particular case, and the condition treated. This provides the facility to undertake various analyses, e.g. the work-load of a consultant, hospital or region by factors such as age, sex, diagnosis, length of stay, death if occurring in hospital, residence of patient, etc. The purpose of HIPE was to provide epidemiological and administrative information for comparative studies of morbidity and resource use and thus to aid hospital service planning. For example, the HIPE can show the age distribution of patients admitted to each specialty, enable waiting times for admission to hospital in various regions to be compared, and provide analyses of discharges and deaths by source of admission.

HIPE data is now selected from Hospital Activity Analysis (HAA) (discussed later) by each region and sent to the Office of Population Censuses and Surveys. Information is published jointly by the DHSS and the Office of Population Censuses and Surveys.[44]

The early faith in the usefulness of this information has been tempered by subsequent criticisms. Forsyth and Logan's suggestion[54] that 'Hospital In-Patient Enquiry avoids all the pitfalls of SH3' is countered by a King's Fund Working Party on the application of economic principles to health service management[1] which states that HIPE 'suffers from the same problem of SH3 in that it is event- rather than patient-oriented.' Other criticisms include:

1. Conceived as a source of information about morbidity, it is deficient in that only a selected fraction of diseases require admission to hospital.

2. The accuracy of the information collected has been shown to be deficient, particularly for diagnosis. Note that a Ministry of Health circular[105] stated that 'it should normally be possible for a clerical officer to complete the forms from the medical records without consulting the medical staff.' Williams[144] quotes from a Scottish report discussing 'how females suffered from diseases of the male genital tract and males from diseases of the female genital tract, and how males also seemed to be afflicted with complications of pregnancy, and old people

with diseases of the newborn; and there is no reason to believe that these difficulties of compilation are peculiar to Scotland!'

3. Whilst the sampling rules are clear, there have been occasions when they have not always been consistently applied.

4. Publication of national figures has usually been two years after the event and this, combined with the factor of deficiencies in the 10% sample, means that such information is not useful locally either in terms of administrative or clinical management.

Despite these criticism, HIPE has a number of valuable, if limited, applications. Ramsay[119] has shown how and to what extent HIPE can be used in planning, and demonstrations of changes in and differences between utilisation of facilities and changes in practice trends are readily available. Examples include changes in admission patterns for different diseases over time and between regions,[12 18] differences in length of patient stay patterns[9 69] and patterns of bed use by diagnostic groups.[8]

## Hospital Activity Analysis

By 1969, the deficiencies of HIPE for local hospital use were widely accepted and directly referred to in the Department of Health and Social Security (DHSS) Memorandum HM(69) 79[38] which stated that 'the management of the hospital service increasingly demands better factual information in order to make the best use of scarce resources.' HAA was specifically introduced to combat the perceived and actual inadequacies of SH3 and HIPE information. The system, described by Benjamin[15] and Rowe and Brewer[125], requires the collection of information about every discharge from acute hospitals in England and Wales. As with HIPE the introduction of the system was phased, but virtually all general hospitals in the country are now covered. The Scottish equivalent system is entitled Scottish Hospital In-Patient Statistics and is described by Parkin *et al.*[116] HAA normally excludes the specialties of obstetrics and psychiatry but psychiatry has a separate data collection method (Mental Health Enquiry) and both specialties are covered by HIPE.

HAA information is usually abstracted from the case notes and, as with HIPE, information is collected about the patient, his condition, operation, if any, and other administrative data (comprehensive list in HM(69) 79).[38] Some regions collect a carbon copy of the top sheet in the case notes (Form HMRI) in the hope that this will give a greater degree of accuracy than the abstraction method. This system is not always popular because of the design of Form HMRI. Provision is made for the collection of additional items of interest to a particular consultant, hospital or region. Such information can be incorporated provided it is expressed in quantitative or numerically coded terms, e.g. number of blood transfusions, severity of condition, or type of x-ray. The completion of the forms can be a combined effort and can involve clerks, secretaries, nurses and doctors but is more usually left to clerical staff. The forms are generally transported to regional centres and punched for computer analysis. Certain validation procedures are carried out by most regions (e.g. searching for male gynaecology cases, paediatric cases over 15 years of age, or patients under 60 in the geriatric specialty) and some users perform their own validation checks, both before submitting HMRI forms and on receipt of analyses (e.g. cross-checks with other data bases). HAA was intended to provide doctors and administrators at hospital and regional level with an information system in which details relating to individual patients were brought together. This was to be done at low cost with rapid retrieval and minimal disturbance in collection. It was hoped to engage the interest of doctors and administrators by giving them clear, well-thought-out analyses with brief commentaries indicating the salient facts, thus enabling the better use of resources and aiding long-term planning and day-to-day management. At the same time, this information base would yield the 10% sample for HIPE.

As with HIPE, initial optimism has been tempered by later criticisms and, in the case of HAA, there has been so much criticism that confidence in it is currently very low. Among the criticisms are:

1. The information collected is not sufficiently comprehensive, there is a lack of integration with other sources, and the outcome of patient care is unknown. Routinely there is no resource usage recorded other than beds; there is a paucity of clinical information in that only international disease labels and operation labels are recorded; the system remains case-oriented rather than patient-oriented; and there is a need to link the information with other health data. The absence of information about the increasing use of out-patient facilities for minor surgery, endoscopy, chemotherapy, etc. reduces considerably the value of information about bed use.

2. The quantity and format of the information presented has not secured an enthusiastic response from clinicians and administrators and there is a constant plea for routine presentation to be severely restricted, with concentration on small amounts of immediately relevant information.

3. The accuracy and completeness of the information chosen for collection is doubted by many. Such doubts were beautifully expressed in the British Medical Journal correspondence column by Rohde[122] when he reported that his latest batch of HAA was 'grossly inaccurate; the number of patients recorded as leaving in this quarter was exactly half those I myself had noted. Even more alarming was a letter accompanying the statistics saying: "Increased accuracy is now being achieved and we are rapidly approaching the stage where the figures can be used at local and regional level for managerial and epidemiological purposes."' Rohde's sentiments find considerable support amongst clinicians, administrators and researchers. The Royal Commission on the NHS[124] discovered that a region which had validated its HAA data had discovered a 30% error rate but that 'this finding was neither formally communicated to the medical records staff responsible for HAA, nor was it recorded to warn future users of these data – because it was thought that this would undermine the credibility of HAA.' The few studies published on completeness and accuracy demonstrate varying results – from 'gross deficiency' to 'almost as good as the case notes'.[86 87 97 100 117]

4. The feedback of HAA has been slow and, whilst the lag varies between regions and over time, it has taken as long as two years and is seldom less then six weeks. The delays often commence at the hospital when doctors fail to complete discharge summaries, but they can occur at all stages of the process between collection of information and presentation of analyses.

In spite of such criticisms, HAA has its disciples. It is not always possible to gather from published documents the exact extent to which HAA is 'used' as opposed to being 'potentially useful'. Some of the uses include:

1. Measuring and describing activities such as use of resources and analysis of length of stay patterns.[761]

2. An information base for a diagnostic index,[86 130 142] and outcome studies.[770]

3. Confirmation and guidance in decision-making, e.g. simulation as done by Morris and Handyside with HIPE,[109] and in planning guidelines.[96 141]

## *Ad hoc* Studies

A large number of *ad hoc* studies are referred to throughout this book. Some of the more substantial studies include the work of Meredith *et al.*[104] in analysing bed use by patient dependency, the investigation of the peculiarities of the Liverpool region's allocation of beds summarised by Logan *et al.*,[88] and the work of the Institute for Operational Research and other OR researchers which appear in the publications by Luck *et al.*[91] and Hicks.[72]

## General Comments On Information Sources

SH3, HIPE and HAA have each had approximately a decade in which to be conceived, introduced and criticised. If the cycle is to continue, we are due for the introduction of a new system and indeed the DHSS is currently reviewing information collection, presentation and use in the National Health Service. If we have anything to learn from history, it should be that new systems are not always the greener grass on the other side of the hill; perhaps we should put more effort into improving the accuracy and use of our existing systems. For the reader who had a few doubts about NHS information, this chapter has probably convinced him that any further study is worthless. So let me try to produce some encouragement to proceed. Firstly, this rather critical appraisal of information sources needs to be put into perspective. International comparisons made by Kozak[84] show that, whilst researchers and health service staff in Britain find much to criticise in their information bases, there are many positive attributes. Information is available throughout the country, the variety and detail of information collected is as great as, or greater than, in other countries and, although questions about the quality of the data can be asked of every system, at least Britain has mounted studies of these problems and continually sought to make improvements. Secondly, generalisations about accuracy and quality mask the wide variation from locality to locality. Many hospitals have excellent information systems and show that very many of the criticisms can be overcome. Generalised smears about the inadequacy of data too often conceal an unwillingness to spend time and effort putting things right. Finally, there is increasing evidence, e.g. Yates,[151] that hospital data, particularly when used for large-scale comparisons, can highlight genuine and significant differences in practice between hospitals and specialties despite the inherent inaccuracies it contains.

# 4

# *Dare we use the information?*

DIFFICULTIES IN INTERPRETING RESULTS.

The tasks of making a diagnosis and choosing appropriate treatment can be aided by various forms of measurement, but at the same time complexity creeps in. Common problems of measurement include:

1. The need to ensure that measurements are correct. In medicine this involves the identification and control of errors in observation and machine analysis.

2. The necessity to make value judgements in interpreting results. A haemoglobin level of 17 may or may not be significant, even if it has been accurately measured. The establishment of a 'normal' range requires a value judgement.

3. Some measurements may indicate that something is wrong, but not what is wrong. Very few tests are specific for aetiology.

4. Information is required not only of the result but also of the conditions under which the measurement was made. A plasma cortisol level in isolation is of no value for diagnostic purposes unless the time and conditions of collection are known.

5. The volume and range of results available can confuse rather than clarify the problem. Biochemical and haematological profiles are not universally accepted as valuable assets.

Interpreting results in management presents many similar problems. If anything it is more complex because there is no single decision-maker. This chapter discusses the choice and presentation of information in the light of inaccuracies of fact and uncertainties of value judgement.

Willingly or otherwise, doctors take part in decision-making processes regarding the use of resources. Often they feel that these processes are inept and time-consuming, but on the other hand they are afraid to leave such decisions to bodies which have no medical advice. It is a 'Catch 22' situation for the doctor who has to forsake time spent on 'his' patients in order to try to defend their interest or improve their prospects. Doctors believe that, unless the medical viewpoint and value judgements are included, then the decisions made will not be sound, nor will commitment to those decisions be assured. The difficulties of their situation are compounded by the use of some of the quantified data referred to in Chapter 3. Doctors can be in the uneasy situation where their sense of what is factual is at variance with the quantitative data provided. In such circumstances there is a need for some practising clinicians to devote time to understanding the characteristics of the information available so that they can guide those concerned with the choice and presentation of that information. It is not satisfactory to leave the subject to the care of medical records staff, administrators and management scientists. One advantage likely to accrue from the attention of practising clinicians is that they can advise on the type of information and form of presentation that is required and understood by their medical colleagues. There are well-developed skills and methods of presentation used in the teaching of medicine for undergraduate and postgraduate purposes, some of which can be usefully transferred to management situations. Another advantage is that clinicians provide an independent check on the accuracy, completeness, and relevance of the information – not all administrators are renowned for presenting well-chosen and accurate information!

## The Choice Of Information

When analysing a situation for oneself it is desirable to have information which is accurate, complete and relevant. Accuracy and completeness are mostly matters of fact whilst relevance is wholly a matter of judgement.

### Accuracy and completeness
Errors can occur at the point of collection, during analysis and upon presentation. This section concentrates on the identification and reduction of errors at the point of collection. In using the words 'accuracy' and 'completeness', I distinguish between making a correct or incorrect

observation (accuracy) and failing or not failing to make that observation (completeness). This distinction is not, however, sufficient for the purposes of identifying the types and sources of errors. Ackoff and Emery[2] suggest that three types of error occur when collecting information. Observational errors can be made through *systematic distortion, fog,* and *mirage.* Let me try to illustrate each of these types by giving examples from hospitals.

With *systematic distortion,* no information is lost but rather it is changed in an orderly or systematic way. Systematic distortion is typified by the behaviour of a clerical officer who was responsible for collecting HIPE information about the discharges in a small hospital. The clerk did not adhere to the 1-in-10 sample method outlined but would always select discharges with a familiar diagnosis (for which he knew the ICD code number) in order to save time in referring to the International Classification of Diseases references books.

In *fog,* some information is partly or completely hidden or lost. HAA clerks who have the responsibility of observing and recording diagnostic information frequently find themselves confronted by a fog of voluminous, badly-filed and poorly-written case notes. In such circumstances, they may fail to record a secondary or complicating diagnosis and information may thus be lost.

The third type of error is called *mirage.* In this case something that is not present is imagined and added to the information. In a situation where a late-afternoon bed state is being collected, some ward staff and junior doctors attempt to defend their ward from a busy night of admissions. With the knowledge that checks will not be made, the returning message states that all beds are full – empty beds are filled with imaginary patients.

The three types of error described can be further subdivided into four sources of error. At the risk of providing too much detail, I would suggest that Ackoff and Emery's classification can aid both our understanding and identification of errors. Their four sources of error are in the observer, the observed, the instruments used, and in the environment. This classification will be familiar to medical scientists. In each of the types of error illustrated above, the errors were basically those of the observers. Errors are sometimes created by the person who is being observed. In interview situations, the interviewee may lie consistently (systematic distortion), talk ambiguously (fog), or describe events which never occurred (mirage). In the type of quantitative information bases used in hospital management this source of error is rarely of interest but must be considered when looking at sources of attitude survey data, e.g. patient satisfaction surveys, or when analysing patient-reported symptoms in case notes.

Instrument errors are well known in medical science (e.g. a sphygmo-manometer consistently under-recording blood pressure) and although, in management, instruments ranging from the typewriter to a computer are used, I would wish to broaden the definition of 'instruments' to include 'systems'. SH3 guidelines and ICD code books are some of the manager's instruments. Systematic distortion occurs when inadequate definitions are chosen. Until 1963, rheumatology was not separately recorded on SH3 forms, but we cannot conclude that no rheumatology was undertaken before that date. Fog distortion is illustrated by the use of midnight bed occupancy counts which fail to identify patients who do not stay overnight. SH3 guidelines at one time regarded the allocated beds for a period to be determined by the number of beds allocated at the end of the period. On the occasions when this figure was higher than the average allocation for the period, it would produce a mirage of beds that never existed.

Errors caused by the environment are probably not a significant factor when studying HAA and SH3 information (as compared with air-temperature changes in certain medical measurements) but a busy office can create noise and pressures that result in both fog and mirage effects.

Table 2 illustrates some of the types and sources of error which can occur in the collection of information and the classification may provide some guidance to the detection of errors. In practice, the most important sources of error in the collection of hospital bed statistics lie within the 'observer' and 'instrument' categories. Instrument errors tend to be consistent and fairly easily detected but observer errors are far more difficult to identify and correct. The rest of this section concentrates on the reduction of observer errors.

Complete elimination of error is seldom possible, often expensive, and sometimes not necessary. Greater accuracy and completeness can be attained in hospital information systems by:

1. Occasional duplication of information collection and subsequent analysis.
2. Regular comparisons between different sources of information.
3. Creating an environment in which interest and encouragement is shown to those staff who have the difficult and unexciting task of collecting information (which probably implies frequent and noticed use of the information they collect).

*Table 2*
**Examples of sources and types of errors of observation**

|  | Systematic distortion | Fog | Mirage |
|---|---|---|---|
| Observer | Clerk who chooses HIPE sample on the basis of patients with an easily coded diagnosis | The difficulties of finding information because of voluminous and badly filed notes | Pretending a ward is full of patients in order to avoid receiving admissions |
| Observed | Mainly only important when analysing patient reported symptoms in case notes or when studying patient-attitude surveys *e.g.* lie consistently | *e.g.* talk ambiguously | *e.g.* Make up events |
| Instrument | 'Poor' definitions in SH3 guidelines and in ICD and operation codes | Midnight count failing to identify certain patients who stay overnight | Old SH3 ruling on bed complements could give higher than actual complement |
| Environment | – | Office noise | Office noise |

4. Arranging adequate education and training of all staff involved.
5. Shortening the line of communication between the points of collection, analysis and use.

The following three case studies attempt to illustrate the first three recommendations listed above. Each case study is produced to show the methods used rather than the results obtained.

*Duplicate checking*

CASE STUDY

Information from HAA sources was used by the author and a consultant physician to identify 140 cases discharged under the care of seven physicians. For each case, the HAA information retrieved was case-note number, name, age, admission and discharge dates, and diagnoses. Each day the medical records department obtained the first fifteen case notes listed for one consultant. If a case note was not available, the reason was noted and a case note selected from the reserve list of five. The author checked all information except diagnostic information for fifteen case notes in less than half an hour and, the next morning, with the physician reading the case notes, established what diagnosis had been recorded and whether it matched the HAA statement of diagnosis. This procedure also took less than half an hour and the case notes were returned to the medical records department by 9.00 a.m. It was necessary to use the reserve list of case notes on 23 occasions but always there was a valid reason for non-availability (e.g. patient re-admitted to same or other hospital, case notes on way to or from out-patient department). In considering the patient, administrative and diagnostic information comparisons were made between the HAA print-out and case sheet forms (which were not part of the documentation sent for coding). No errors were found in case note numbers, spelling of names, sex, and date of admission. On one occasion the patient's age was incorrectly recorded, and on two occasions age was omitted. Eight differences in discharge date were noted. Five of the eight appeared to be a difference of only one day but it was common for case note information to be internally inconsistent. For diagnostic information the discharge letter was used as the primary check document but, once again, diagnostic recording was not always internally consistent with case notes. In no case did the diagnosis shown on the HAA print-out differ from the discharge letters. One source of error was detected in that there were cases when ICD classification separated a diagnosis into two categories (e.g. thyrotoxicosis with or without mention of goitre) and this classification was not always known by the doctor who simply recorded thyrotoxicosis. This led to an incorrect coding of the actual diagnosis, although a faithful recording of the discharge letter diagnosis. Eight instances of this nature were discovered. In the case of second and complicating diagnosis no errors of commission were made, although a number of errors of omission were noted. The conclusion reached by the investigators and the division of medicine concerned was that a high degree of accuracy could be attributed to the information available from HAA in general medicine in that particular hospital and that the information base could be used with confidence.

Duplicate checking of information is both time-consuming and expensive and must be considered impracticable on a continuing basis. Duplication on a selected basis can help to improve and maintain standards. The published surveys of accuracy and completeness referred to in Chapter 3, and other unpublished studies, have shown that the information most susceptible to error in HAA is diagnosis and operation.

*Comparisons between different sources*
To obtain a 100% complete HAA data base usually means delaying the analysis of a large amount of information in order to wait for a small number of forms. Frequently, to avoid delay, a small percentage of information is disregarded. The question raised is how typical of the total are the 90–95% of HAA returns, and whether an incomplete sample can be used to analyse bed usage between wards and specialties without the worry of the peculiarities of the final small percentage. No overall answer can be given to this question as there are considerable differences within and between hospitals and specialties over time. A number of unpublished surveys have shown that the last small percentage can include high proportions of discharges from particular specialties, high numbers of long-stay patients and a large proportion of complex multi-diagnosis cases.

CASE STUDY
A surgical division used HAA information to analyse retrospectively bed use on three general surgical wards. The general surgeons then moved on to simulate different emergency admission patterns in order to assess the effect of those patterns on overall bed use. The consultants were aware that approximately 97% of discharges were included in the data base but, as the mean length of stay for those cases was comparable with the overall figure, they considered 97% completeness to be satisfactory. Pleased with the results of the emergency pattern simulation, they decided to use the data base to make a detailed study of deaths on surgical wards. The requested print-out was returned and, to their disbelief, there were no surgical deaths. Investigations showed that the death case notes were all sent to the postgraduate centre for a quarterly deaths conference and were never returned to the records department for the abstraction of HAA information. One hundred percent completeness was not essential for one study but vital for another.

The doubts raised about the completeness of HAA information led the hospital staff to request an analysis of the number of cases discharged by each specialty over one year. The results were compared with SH3 returns and HAA discharges and ranged from 65–104% of SH3 records. Attempts to match the two figures highlighted errors not only in HAA completeness but also in certain inaccuracies in the definition of day-case and one-day-stay patients. The checking helped to identify which specialties had a poor record for returning diagnostic summaries and encouraged the hospital to ensure a match of 98–100% before using HAA information. After three years' checking, the hospital was able to report that, when reviewing a year's work in the March of the following year, there were no discharge summaries missing for the review year.

## *The importance of interest and commitment*

CASE STUDY
A division of obstetrics and gynaecology, drawing on the experience of work done elsewhere, concentrated on examining diagnostic and operation information. The selection of case notes was made in such a way as to divide doctor- and clerk-completed summaries and also to study what proportion of summary sheets were amended by the coding clerk (because of obvious errors) before transmission to the computer. Only 50 case notes were studied. No errors in the record of first operation were discovered and in one case the second operation was omitted. In the case of diagnoses the results were so appalling that the intended survey of 100 case notes was terminated when 50 notes had been completed; 19 of the 50 had incorrectly recorded diagnoses. After routine checking by the coding clerk, this number was reduced to 11. Doctor-completed summaries were more accurate than clerk-completed summaries but eight doctors' errors in 25 seemed unacceptable. (Other studies have shown clerical staff to be more accurate than doctors in recording information on diagnostic summaries.) In the hospital studied, the completion of diagnostic summaries had always been poor. The division concerned had never previously requested any HAA information and there was some evidence to suggest that the consultants were unaware that the information was collected. Month by month over three successive years the hospital's performance in returning diagnostic summaries had been very poor (83–87%).

The sudden interest of the division in the HAA information, and the process of checking that information, coincided with a striking improvement in the completeness and accuracy of the information. The completeness of returns immediately rose to over 95% and the hospital soon led the district in completion rates.

My observations suggest that, whilst error rates vary enormously from place to place and from time to time in the same place, better results are almost always obtained when the local checking of records is accompanied by direct interest shown in the staff who collect them.

## Relevance

Accuracy and completeness are easy to define and check by comparison with the subject of relevance. Many of us have a tendency to feel that our thoughts and actions are more 'relevant' than those of our colleagues. Judgements about relevance are made when defining the problems at hand, in choosing the information we need, and in selecting the measures we use. A study of in-patient waiting lists raises many questions which need judgements of relevance. Does a waiting list reflect real need? Should the study be of patient numbers, patient waiting time, or both? Should the study examine patients who are waiting or those who have waited? Which measure of waiting time should be used – arithmetic mean, median, or some other measure?

Differing judgements about relevance can be illustrated by looking at the use of bed occupancy. Year after year, in spite of criticisms particularly from medical and nursing staff, the term 'bed occupancy' has been employed when discussing the performance of hospitals. The first Cogwheel Reports[106] stated that 'Administrators (and others) often tend to give undue weight to occupancy figures. As a result, patients may occasionally be kept in hospital for longer than necessary out of a misplaced desire to improve occupancy figures regardless of the adverse effect on turnover and actual bed use, and with no consideration for the desire of the patient to return home as quickly as possible.' Williams[144] says, 'There is a vast difference between a bedstead and a bed with adequate staff and services. A high bed occupancy rate may be associated with poor medical practice and service to the community.' Clinicians, however, fall into the trap themselves. Gardiner and Moreny[58] suggest that 75% occupancy is a 'safe figure' at which to run surgical wards and that above that it becomes unsafe for reasons of cross-infection. Administrators' worry about bed occupancy is summed up by Griffiths[64] who says that 'occupancy is frequently uncontrolled ... administrators seem to regard it as evidence of divine providence rather than of good managerial performance.' Sometimes not only the concept but the figures themselves are misunderstood. A community health council sought an explanation from an area health authority about an 80% bed occupancy and were assured by the AHA that such an occupancy was 'usual'. 'But when the council examined the statistics they found a very different picture and discovered that in some cases almost one in five beds were empty every day'.[71] Bed occupancy is an unsuitable measure for comparing units or for assessing performance over a period of time. Firstly, it combines and confuses two elements: the number of patients admitted, and how long those patients stay. Two adjacent 30-bedded medical wards may each have an occupancy of 85% while one ward admits twice the number of patients as its counterpart during the same period of time. Secondly, bed occupancy takes no account of what happens to the patient in hospital or after discharge. Length of stay is influenced by differences in case-mix, staff availability, the quantity, availability and balance of support services (e.g. radiology, pathology, domestics), staff training, teaching commitments, home nursing availability, and general practitioner cover. In spite of this we still use the measure throughout the country from divisions to DHSS and we have very different perceptions of its relevance.

Relevance relates essentially to the place, the people, the time, and the situation. Getting relevance 'right' can be aided by obtaining the views of others in order to get additional perspectives against which to balance one's own judgements. Another aid to securing agreement with others on relevance is to ensure that, in communicating with them, one builds from their existing knowledge the facts and concepts one is trying to communicate. Adults prefer to relate new information to their existing knowledge and, if they are unable to do so, newly presented information may be dismissed as irrelevant.

## The Presentation Of Information

Securing the commitment of others to take action can be aided or hindered by the form of presentation. It is not sufficient for information to be of satisfactory accuracy, completeness and relevance – it must also be seen to be so by the recipient. The recipient's confidence can be built, not upon the fact that the information is totally accurate, complete and relevant (which is seldom possible), but on the fact that it is usable. Often the discipline and honesty of admitting the type and magnitude of any errors helps to create confidence in the information.

Having chosen accurate, complete and relevant information the presentation needs to be understandable, acceptable, timely, appropriate in quantity, and to have a certain originality. These five characteristics are matters of value judgement and on occasions they may contradict one another as well as the basic characteristics of accuracy, completeness and relevance. It is very common to find that complete information is only available at the sacrifice of timeliness and that accurate information is not acceptable.

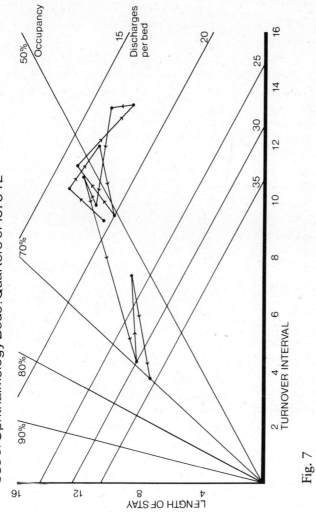

Fig. 7

### Monthly Admissions to Acute Psychiatric Beds in a Hospital 1976-78

a.Presented as a RAILWAY TIMETABLE

|      | J  | F  | M  | A  | M  | J  | J  | A  | S  | O  | N  | D  |
|------|----|----|----|----|----|----|----|----|----|----|----|----|
| 1976 | 41 | 45 | 40 | 41 | 42 | 42 | 40 | 40 | 47 | 34 | 34 | 38 |
| 1977 | 37 | 34 | 36 | 38 | 27 | 35 | 39 | 23 | 30 | 27 | 34 | 38 |
| 1978 | 31 | 24 | 27 | 32 | 29 | 18 | 14 | 28 | 27 | 32 | 31 | 39 |

b.Presented as a GRAPH

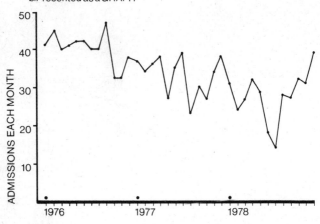

Fig. 8

## Understandability

Complete understanding involves receiving and comprehending the information presented. Information is usually received verbally, on paper, or by some other form of visual display. Despite the obvious need to ensure that information is received, health service management continues to be a haven of photostat copies that cannot be read, speakers at meetings who fail to face their audience and to speak in an audible fashion, and visual aids which are upside down, back to front, or unreadable from a distance. Reference to the literature (e.g. Calnan and Barabas, [25][26] Hawkins[67]) can be of aid to the presenters of information.

Even when information is received there is no guarantee of comprehension. Figure 7 can be criticised on presentational grounds for attempting to convey too much information but, more important, the circumstances in which such a diagram is used are crucial. The tech-

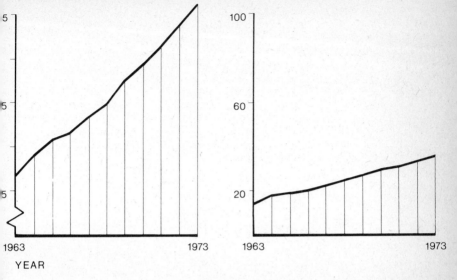

Pathology Requests (in 00,000) for a Region 1963-1973

Fig. 9

nique developed by Barber and Johnson[11] is of value to the receiver only when he has studied the variables displayed and the methods used. Comprehension requires certain existing levels of knowledge, familiarity, and common language, which may have to be built up over a period of time. (An explanation of Fig. 7 and the technique used appears in the Appendix.)

Both receipt and comprehension of numerical information can be aided by the use of graphs. The difference between the 'railway timetable' type of presentation and graphical presentation is illustrated in Fig. 8. Many feel that the significance of the information is more readily seen at a glance by viewing the graph rather than the figures. It also has to be recognised that some fear the god, 'number', and others merely have marked preference for visual presentation (photograph of model compared with statistical description 36–22–36). Graphs can however be distorted by cunning use of scales in order to portray value judgements. Figure 9 shows constant and dramatic growths in pathology test requests.

## Acceptability

Truth can sometimes be painful and there are occasions on which it is not only kinder but wiser not to present information which makes a recipient strongly defensive and uncooperative. Comparative work-load figures often come into this category.

CASE STUDY

A group of consultants who felt their specialty was under pressure were surprised to discover that the number of discharges per bed (throughput) was lower than that of their colleagues in nearby hospitals. That fact alone was difficult enough to swallow at one time. A demonstration that the lower throughput was achieved in circumstances generally considered to be more favourable (i.e. a lower proportion of elderly admissions) stretched the acceptability of the information presented (see Fig. 10). In this instance the information was presented at two separate meetings – two months apart.

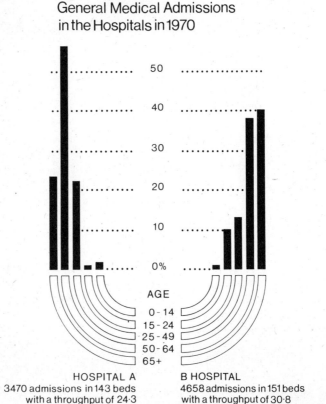

Fig. 10

There are occasions when some information is best withheld for a period of time to enable recipients to accustom themselves to the difference between their perceptions of the situation and someone else's description of it. To secure acceptability one sometimes not only withholds information, one distorts it.

CASE STUDY
The chairman of a working party set up to examine the falling workload of a hospital drafted a letter which sought the views of all clinical staff on the reasons for the steadily falling work-load. In the letter he pointed out that the trend had changed in recent months and that a slight increase in patient numbers had occurred. The working party suggested that the figures did not support the statement made (i.e. no recent increase had occurred) but agreed with the chairman that if the co-operation of the staff was to be obtained it would be necessary to make such a statement.

Clinicians know only too well the dilemma of presenting unwelcome clinical information. Should it be given to the patient all at once, a little at a time, or not at all? It is a difficult judgement to determine how much, if any, withholding or distortion of information is desirable in order to protect and support views and prejudices.

## Timeliness
It has been said that the best available information at the right time has ten times the value of all the information presented too late. Speed is perceived by many doctors and administrators at hospital level as being of great importance. The absence of information is a regular excuse for failure to act.

CASE STUDY
The doctors and administrators at one hospital struggled to achieve a high standard of accuracy and completeness in the production of HAA forms. The failure of the regional authority to analyse and return information within six to nine months was seen by the hospital staff to be the chief hindrance in the use of the information to improve utilisation of the wards. They required immediate analyses of changing trends in occupancy, admission rates, and diagnostic mix, in order to reallocate their resources and HAA singularly failed to meet that requirement.

On the other hand the few hospitals which have systems with the capacity to produce relatively instant information appear to be shy of making use of such good fortune.

CASE STUDY
In another hospital, HAA data was collected daily on both the admission and discharge of patients. The availability of a computer on site enabled the analysis and print-out of information such as admission and discharge dates, source of admission and discharge, and patients' age and sex. For every ward or specialty, detailed analyses were available twenty-four hours after the event and yet in five years there had been no request for such information on any time-scale of less than one month. When information was eventually produced for divisional meetings on the time scale of one week, the usual reaction to any movement or trend was 'wait and see'.

Perhaps the most important reason for achieving a speedy analysis and presentation of information is that it does not enable the criticism of poor timeliness to be made.

## Quantity

Attenders at meetings are notorious for explaining how little time there is to read the enormous amounts of literature and data with which they are confronted. Even outside formal meetings, those concerned with operational management, whether clinical or administrative, find they have little time to sift through vast quantities of information. Selection of material in such circumstances is essential. The use of exception reporting mechanisms[149] and such methods as cumulative sum techniques[53 147] can reduce quantity, although the work involved in determining the criteria against which exceptions will be selected can be very time-consuming in itself.

CASE STUDY
A hospital faced with a declining use of beds formed a group of medical, nursing and administrative staff to examine the problem and initiate action to reduce the number of empty beds. The group took action which it felt would increase the number of patients admitted to the hospital and set expected criteria in terms of the numbers of planned and emergency admissions, age range of admissions, number of inter-ward transfers, number of extra beds, length of stay patterns, number of empty beds, etc., for all specialties and the whole hospital. The review of these criteria on a quarterly basis normally involved the study of hundreds of figures, but by prospectively agreeing expected performance the number of 'significant' (i.e. important in the opinion of the group) items was reduced considerably. Figure 11 illustrates for one criterion the data used to help determine the standard and the actual performance against that standard.

## Originality

The commercial and advertising world places much emphasis on unusual and original presentation. Even in hospital management there is a place for originality. As mentioned earlier, the use of a graph in a situation which traditionally uses railway timetable type of statistical reports has been known to inspire even clinicians to examine the basic data. A further example is that the constant use of bed occupancy figures over the last few years has not only built up an immunity to a 'bad' measure but also stifled the willingness to study the use of hospital beds. Transferring attention to bed emptiness has sometimes overcome such reluctance.

CASE STUDY
The presentation of 'empty bed' graphs and figures has been observed to produce more response and impact than bed occupancy figures. One hospital secretary who had empty bed charts (e.g. Fig. 12) displayed in his office found that he had to move them to another location after four weeks because of the frequent interruptions of consultants and other senior staff. A medical executive committee uninterested in a 75% bed occupancy was provoked into action on discovering that there were on average over 100 empty beds in the hospital. As the hospital had 600 beds, one might have expected the committee to appreciate that 75% meant 150 empty beds!

This chapter has outlined eight characteristics concerning the choice and presentation of information. This is an entirely personal view of the characteristics. If I were to add another to my list it would be that of 'incompleteness'! No self-respecting group of information receivers wants its work done for it. Presented information should lead to action, not pre-empt it.

Percentage of Empty Beds in a District General Hospital 1964-1976 (quarters)

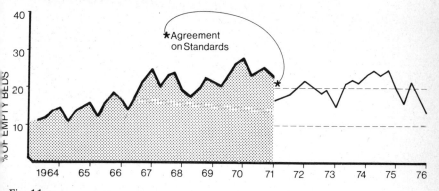

Fig. 11

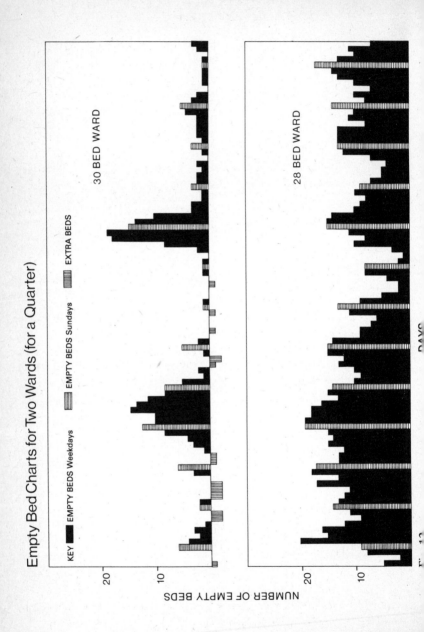

Empty Bed Charts for Two Wards (for a Quarter)

# 5

# *Can the information identify problems?*

## DIAGNOSTIC INVESTIGATION

Each clinician has his own investigating style. There are variations in the amount of emphasis placed on observation of and discussion with the patient and the extent, order, and timing of routine and special investigations. Individual managers and groups of managers also vary in their approaches to identifying problems, and investigation can be mounted at various levels from the local hospital to the regional health authority.

This chapter outlines some methods of investigating the provision, use, and spare capacity of beds which can be undertaken at a local level.

---

Investigation of bed allocation and use ranges from small studies of an individual consultant's patients to international comparisons of the performance of whole countries' hospital stock. Ths book chooses to concentrate on examining bed use at the level of a large hospital or group of hospitals within a district. Studies at this level can be personal and it is relatively easy to obtain the commitment of the individual medical staff involved in a way which is not always possible in more widely-based studies. At hospital level the data base is usually large enough to provide at least some comparative study and thus stimulate discussion and further enquiries. One major advantage of choosing larger hospitals or groups of smaller hospitals in comparison with individual wards or specialities is that there is a greater possibility of arranging 'trade-offs' between areas of relative deficiency or surplus of bed provision.

## Internal Comparisons

SH3 information for a five-year period can provide a rough but useful guide to bed availability and use. The presentation of the information on Barber–Johnson[11] diagrams can help identify trends and isolate areas for further examination. As this chapter makes considerable use of this technique, readers who are unfamiliar with the work of Barber and Johnson are advised to study the Appendix before proceeding. To illustrate this type of comparison let us consider the figures from a district, for one year only. District A is fictitious only in order to provide anonymity for the hospitals and specialties concerned and to simplify presentation. None of the individual figures presented are fictitious – they come from specialties in three districts.

### District A

District A is in the heart of a city and there is a considerable overlap of patient flow between adjacent districts. This means that the district general hospital does not provide a complete service for its whole district population, some specialty requirements being met by other districts. The district general hospital has developed over a period of time on a workhouse site and future developments include provision of an obstetric unit and psychiatric and geriatric assessment units. This will lead to the complete closure of the maternity hospital. The bed emptiness in the district general hospital is 23%. This is lower than the national average for acute hospitals but typical of district general hospital sites.

Table 3 shows some of the basic statistics for 1977. Available and occupied beds, discharges and deaths, and waiting lists, are all recorded at hospital level on SH3 forms. Mean length of stay, discharges and deaths per bed (throughput), turnover interval and percentage emptiness can all be calculated from the first three columns (see Appendix for calculations). The individual acute specialty figures for the general and maternity hospitals are plotted on a Barber–Johnson diagram (Fig. 13).

The table and figure appear to describe a situation where there is considerable pressure on general medicine (1), traumatic and orthopaedic surgery (6) and urology (7), whilst on the other hand there appears to be relative spare capacity in paediatrics (2) and chest diseases (3). The use of the diagram helps to clarify why there might be less concern about a 40% emptiness in ENT (5), compared with a 23%

**Statistics for District A, 1977**

| Specialty | Ref. | Beds Available (AM) | Beds Occupied (AM) | Discharges and deaths | Waiting list nos. | Length of stay (days) (AM) | Discharges and deaths per bed per year (AM) | Turnover internal (days) (AM) | Emptiness (%) (AM) |
|---|---|---|---|---|---|---|---|---|---|
| *General Hospital* | | | | | | | | | |
| General Medicine | 1 | 140·1 | 131·0 | 3997 | — | 12·0 | 28·5 | 0·8 | 7 |
| Paediatrics | 2 | 58·7 | 29·0 | 1135 | — | 9·3 | 19·3 | 9·5 | 51 |
| Chest Diseases | 3 | 219·2 | 153·5 | 2019 | — | 27·8 | 9·2 | 11·9 | 30 |
| General Surgery | 4 | 125·2 | 91·5 | 3689 | 835 | 9·0 | 29·5 | 3·3 | 27 |
| ENT | 5 | 21·7 | 13·1 | 1152 | 407 | 4·1 | 53·1 | 2·7 | 40 |
| Trau. & Orthopaedics | 6 | 94·1 | 91·1 | 2039 | 547 | 16·3 | 21·7 | 0·5 | 3 |
| Urology | 7 | 29·1 | 27·7 | 711 | 168 | 14·2 | 24·4 | 0·7 | 5 |
| Thoracic Surgery | 8 | 41·1 | 31·8 | 801 | 25 | 14·5 | 19·5 | 4·2 | 23 |
| Gynaecology | 9 | 49·9 | 30·0 | 2442 | 212 | 4·5 | 49·0 | 3·0 | 40 |
| | | 779·1 | 598·7 | 17985 | | | 23·1 | | 23 |
| *Maternity Hospital* | | | | | | | | | |
| Obstetrics | 10 | 75·2 | 44·9 | 2604 | — | 6·3 | 34·6 | 4·2 | 40 |
| S.C. Baby Unit | 11 | 15·1 | 11·7 | 351 | — | 12·1 | 23·2 | 3·5 | 23 |
| *Geriatric Hospital* | | | | | | | | | |
| Geriatrics | 12 | 234·6 | 220·8 | 1298 | — | 62·1 | 5·5 | 3·9 | 6 |
| *Psychiatric Hospital* | | | | | | | | | |
| Mental Illness | 13 | 701·2 | 606·7 | 1341 | — | 165·1 | 1·9 | 25·7 | 13 |

AM = Arithmetic Mean
Source: Based on actual figures from the SH3 forms of three districts.

emptiness in thoracic surgery (8). A high turnover interval can be of more concern than a high figure of percentage emptiness.

On face value there would appear to be some scope for a reallocation of beds in order to reduce the pressure for some specialties and reduce apparent waste of resources by others.

This type of general review does not highlight the dysfunctions (diseases) suggested in Chapter 2 precisely, but it can give some indications of where to pursue more detailed investigations. Before doing so, it is essential to make some checks on the accuracy and relevance of the data so far examined. Ideally all figures should be checked against

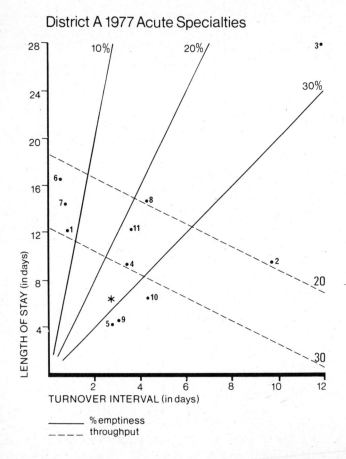

Fig. 13    Source: Table 3

other sources, but this is time-consuming. I would particularly recommend a check of:

1. figures against feelings.
2. relative extremes.
3. bed borrowing figures.
4. the validity of the midnight bed count.
5. the descriptive ability of the arithmetic mean.

Each of these is now examined with particular reference to District A.

### Check figures against feelings
Do the figures presented appear, to those who work in the hospital, to be an adequate description of activity? Inaccurate figures can be identified by presentation to, and discussion with, the staff who work in the units concerned.

> CASE STUDY
> Discussion of the basic figures with members of the hospital's medical committees raised a number of doubts about the accuracy of the data. The most substantial doubts were raised by the medical staff of the maternity hospital about the obstetric figures. After investigation, it transpired that the bed availability figure had been incorrectly recorded. The availability of 75·2 beds was based on a count (now ten years old) which had determined a bed allocation of 80 beds. A number of beds had been closed during the year for upgrading and the number of available bed days lost had been deducted from the original count of 80. Over the last ten years the constant upgrading of the hospital had (through the introduction of more cubicles) reduced the complement to 68 and thus the bed availability figure for the specialty should have been reduced to 63·2 for 1977. The change made to the figures is shown in Table 4. See also the change of position marked * in Fig. 13. The revised figures were consistent with the views held by the obstetricians on work-load. (It was interesting to note that the hospital had chosen to accept a bed complement of 80 when discussing revenue funding with the district and the region, and also when discussing the approval of nurse training schemes with the Central Midwives Board.)

### Check relative extremes
Very high and very low occupancy, throughput, or length of stay are worth a second look, as are figures which change dramatically between two periods of time. Checks of SH3 information are best done by going back to the original returns which are collected on a daily basis at ward level and following their progress through records departments until they appear on SH3 returns. A fund of local interpretations and likely

Table 4
District A obstetric bed use figures, 1977

| | Beds | | Discharges and deaths | Mean length of stay (days) | Discharges and deaths per bed | Turnover Interval (days) | Emptiness % |
|---|---|---|---|---|---|---|---|
| | Available | Occupied | | | | | |
| Original Figures | 75·2 | 44·9 | 2604 | 6·3 | 34·6 | 4·2 | 40 |
| Corrected Figures | 63·2 | 44·9 | 2604 | 6·3 | 41·2 | 2·5 | 29 |

(Note the effect this has on obstetrics (Ref. 10) in Fig. 17.)

sources of error can usually be found. It is often at this stage that the identification of other constraints (e.g. theatres, staffing, revenue) begin to appear. This type of check is by no means foolproof and wild goose chases may be embarked upon because of the use of arithmetic means in the SH3 returns (see below).

### Check bed borrowing figures

The SH3 rules state that, when a bed is borrowed by one specialty, the bed availability of the specialty from which it is borrowed is accordingly reduced and the availability of the borrowing specialty is increased. A simple example illustrates this point. During the winter months the pressure on medicine is such that it is forced to borrow beds from surgery. The number of bed days borrowed during the whole year amounts to 1398. This means that 3·8 available beds (1398/365) are added to medicine and deducted from surgery. Whilst this is a fair way of calculating the figures, two qualifications must be made. Firstly, bed borrowing makes simple data collection more difficult and there is a tendency for inaccuracies to arise. In busy hospitals bed borrowing is not simply between two specialties but between many specialties and includes cross-borrowing; moreover, much of the borrowing is done for only parts of a patient's total stay in hospital. Data collection can thus be a complex procedure for the clerical staff. Secondly, the way in which bed borrowing changes bed availability is slightly artificial. In the example cited above, it is to medicine's advantage (in terms of statistics) to borrow beds at a 100% occupancy. A formal increase in their bed availability by increasing the actual allocation of beds would be unlikely to be followed by a 100% use of those beds. Similarly, beds borrowed from surgery which would not have otherwise been used by the surgeons would have been empty beds. In these circumstances the emptiness figures in surgery appear lower than they might actually have been.

These comments are intended to impress upon investigators the possibility of increased inaccuracies in bed borrowing situations and the slightly false picture of bed use created by bed borrowing (and extra or centre beds).

### Check the validity of the midnight bed count

The use of midnight (i.e. sometime between midnight and 9.00 a.m.) as a census of hospital activity is criticised as being unrepresentative. It does not include patients who are admitted and discharged within twenty-four hours and do not stay over midnight, nor does it include day-cases (which should be counted separately). It is also claimed that it does not always give a true representation of high turnover wards – especially those which frequently admit cases in the mornings and discharge in the afternoons. For such wards, a midday count would reveal a higher figure. Despite these criticisms there has been very little analysis on the subject. The one published paper[36] and other unpublished surveys in district general hospitals have shown that midnight generally underestimates occupancy when compared with either midday or randomly chosen times. The underestimate for most hospitals is generally less than 3%, but in extreme cases the variation ranged from a 2% overestimate to a 10% underestimate. The variation between wards can be greater. My experience is that local checking does not wholly justify the substantial scepticism of midnight counts, but in certain circumstances (e.g. high turnover short-stay wards) care must be taken in interpreting the data.

## Check the descriptive ability of the arithmetic mean

The four variables portrayed on the Barber–Johnson diagram are all average figures. The average used is the arithmetic mean and, whilst there is some value in studying the range and median, the most satisfactory check is an examination of the whole distribution of those figures which are to be studied. An arithmetic mean of 50 empty beds does not indicate how often, if ever, all beds were used.

CASE STUDY

Two of the higher bed emptiness figures in District A appear in the paediatric and gynaecology specialties. Before considering reallocation, an analysis of the mean number of empty beds is required. This can easily be done as the figure is derived from the daily 'midnight' occupancy counts. A day-to-day plotting can be made for each ward and/or specialty. Figures 14 and 15 show the daily figure of emptiness for both specialties. The arithmetic mean quite usefully describes the normal situation in the paediatric unit depicted in Fig. 14 and does indicate that discussions about the release of some bed allocation are distinctly possible. Figure 15 on the other hand demonstrates that the arithmetic mean is influenced by a 20-day period (from day 23) which requires some explanation before attempting to negotiate a review of bed allocation. An additional factor is the wide range of bed emptiness (even excluding the 20-day period) which, if dictated by factors such as theatre availability, would make reallocation of beds extremely difficult.

These five checks on the accuracy and relevance of the data available should enable the investigator to move towards a greater understand-

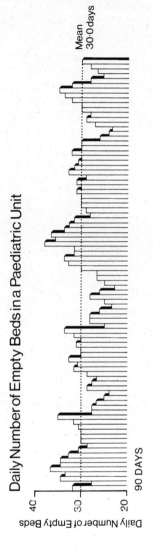

Fig. 14

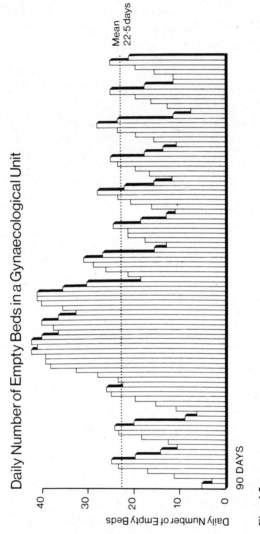

Daily Number of Empty Beds in a Gynaecological Unit

Fig. 15

ing of the problems of allocation and use that exist within his district. It would be advisable to undertake the type of review described above for a three- to five-year period in order to establish trends.

CASE STUDY
Figure 16 shows the five-year pattern of behaviour in the general surgical and general medical specialties of a district general hospital (not District A). In general surgery, activity appears to be constant except for the year of 1975. During this year the three general surgeons adopted an active work to rule policy and the resulting decrease in throughput (and changes in associated measures) can be clearly seen. General medicine

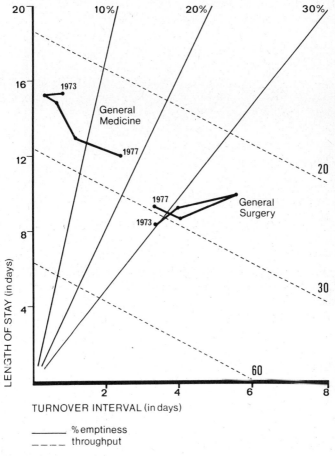

Fig. 16

shows 1973 and 1974 to be years of longer stay and smaller throughput than subsequent years. The explanation in this case is that 1975 saw the appointment of two new physicians who adopted a different policy of activity from that of their predecessors.

In recommending this method of analysing hospital bed statistics, I was initially worried that familiarity with local circumstances enabled an individual to read more into the figures than was justified. In order to test this fear I sought the cooperation of clinicians and administrators in a number of hospitals of which I had no knowledge. I was sent SH3 returns for a five-year period and then undertook an analysis by the method illustrated above and presented the results to the clinicians concerned. The general view of activity was correctly analysed in all but a few cases. In each of these exceptions it transpired that the original data presented had been incorrect. In most hospitals it was even possible to identify with reasonable accuracy which specialties had participated significantly in the 1975 consultants' action. To test the method further, a number of consultants have undertaken this analysis on the work of colleagues in other hospitals. This testing is not of course conclusive but strongly suggests that these so-called 'crude' data are surprisingly sensitive to changes in policy. The reliance of the method on correct bed availability must however be closely watched (see Appendix).

## Inter-district Comparisons

Within a district, comparisons are mainly limited to comparing performance between specialties or comparing one specialty's performance over time. If comparisons are made with other districts a much broader perspective can be gained, but only at the risk of commencing an interminable debate about comparability. For example, look at District B.

### District B
District B serves a town in the heart of a rural area, but the town and much of its surrounding catchment area are within reasonably easy travelling distance of a large city with university and medical school. Patient referral to the university and regional centre hospitals is quite common. Inadequate hospital provision in surrounding areas nevertheless means that for some specialties there is a considerable inflow of patients, which will continue until capital development in surrounding areas is complete in five years' time. The district general hospital feels

itself under considerable pressure and the emptiness of 12%, an average figure for a whole year, is very low (few district general hospitals in this country run at such a low level for a whole year).

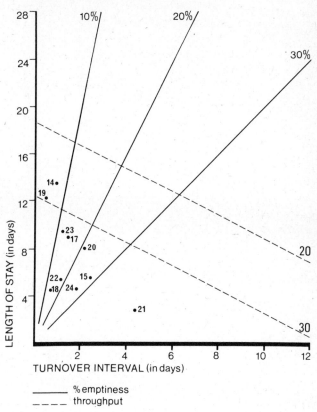

Fig. 17 Source: Table 5

A very different pattern of bed use exists in the acute specialties compared with District A. Table 5 shows that six acute specialties have a turnover interval of less than 1·5 days. The only specialty of Figure 17 that shows a high emptiness of beds is dental surgery[21], which has only 3·4 beds allocated. Unlike District A, there appears to be no scope for internal reallocation of beds between acute specialties and almost certainly District B will be more concerned to study problems of appropriate bed use and examine clinical and administrative policies regarding admission scheduling and discharge. Perhaps the only reallo-

## Table 5
## Statistics for District B, 1977

| Specialty | Ref. | Beds Available (AM) | Occupied (AM) | Discharges and deaths | Waiting list nos. | Length of stay (days) (AM) | Discharges and deaths per bed per year (AM) | Turnover interval (days) (AM) | Emptiness % (AM) |
|---|---|---|---|---|---|---|---|---|---|
| *General Hospital* | | | | | | | | | |
| General Medicine | 14 | 106·2 | 99·3 | 2684 | — | 13·5 | 25·2 | 0·9 | 6 |
| Paediatrics | 15 | 25·0 | 17·4 | 1164 | — | 5·4 | 46·5 | 2·4 | 30 |
| Geriatrics | 16 | 38·0 | 37·2 | 339 | — | 40·1 | 8·9 | 0·9 | 2 |
| General Surgery | 17 | 89·7 | 77·3 | 3242 | 1159 | 8·7 | 36·1 | 1·4 | 14 |
| ENT | 18 | 19·9 | 17·2 | 1430 | 1468 | 4·4 | 71·9 | 0·7 | 14 |
| Trau. & Orthopaedics | 19 | 59·2 | 56·7 | 1740 | 736 | 11·9 | 29·4 | 0·5 | 4 |
| Ophthalmology | 20 | 20·2 | 15·9 | 742 | 349 | 7·8 | 36·8 | 2·1 | 21 |
| Dental Surgery | 21 | 3·4 | 1·3 | 176 | 60 | 2·6 | 51·8 | 4·3 | 62 |
| Gynaecology | 22 | 29·0 | 24·0 | 1705 | 292 | 5·1 | 58·8 | 1·1 | 17 |
| Obstetrics | 23 | 114·2 | 100·9 | 4005 | — | 9·2 | 35·0 | 1·2 | 12 |
| SC Baby Unit | 24 | 22·0 | 15·6 | 1263 | — | 4·5 | 57·4 | 1·8 | 29 |
| Mental Illness | 25 | 30·7 | 25·4 | 391 | — | 23·7 | 12·7 | 4·9 | 17 |
| | | 557·5 | 488·2 | 18881 | | | 34·7 | | 12 |
| *Geriatric Hospital* | | | | | | | | | |
| Geriatrics | 26 | 84·0 | 83·4 | 159 | — | 191·5 | 1·9 | 1·4 | 1 |
| *Mental Handicap Hospital* | | | | | | | | | |
| Mental Handicap | 27 | 587·2 | 537·8 | 156 | — | 1258·3 | 0·2 | 115·5 | 9 |
| *General Practitioner Hospitals* | | | | | | | | | |
| GP 1 | 28 | 21·0 | 18·1 | 224 | — | 29·5 | 10·7 | 4·7 | 14 |
| GP 2 | 29 | 24·0 | 22·5 | 101 | — | 81·3 | 4·2 | 5·4 | 6 |
| GP 3 | 30 | 65·0 | 47·8 | 1953 | 453 | 8·9 | 30·0 | 3·2 | 26 |

AM = Arithmetic Mean
Source: Based on actual figures from the SH3 forms of five districts.

cation of beds based on 1977 patterns lies in a change of use of the GP hospitals.

It is almost impossible to explain the very different performance of Districts A and B with any confidence. Clearly the populations served are different and there may be considerable differences in the amount and quality of hospital service provision and primary care services. Whether such factors could entirely explain differences in performance is difficult to know. Inter-district comparisons can raise some very pointed questions about performance, but at present our range of comparison is frequently too small and we are apt to dismiss differences between neighbouring districts as attributable to some local factors that we alight upon. Current inter-district comparisons are usually confined at best to districts within one region. This limits the number of districts to the range of between 7 and 22. Not only can we jump too quickly to explain inter-district differences, but we can also be unaware

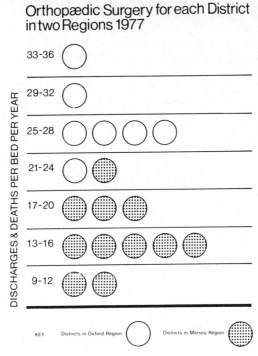

Throughput (Discharges & Deaths per Available Bed) in Traumatic and Orthopædic Surgery for each District in two Regions 1977

Fig. 18   Source: SH 3

of quite significant differences between our local region and other regions. Figure 18 shows the throughput in each of the districts in two regions for trauma and orthopaedic surgery. In each region any district would feel that its throughput was quite normal when compared with that of immediate colleagues, but the national picture would display very wide differences. Inter-district comparisons are now available from the Health Services Management Centre of the University of Birmingham, which enable each district to compare its provision of resources and activity with that of all districts in England. Each district can identify its performance on a distribution (e.g. Fig. 19) and information can be summarised on a profile by means of the conversion of each distribution into a percentile bar (Fig. 20). The resulting profiles (Fig. 21), together with the type of scattergrams illustrated in the Appendix (Fig. H) should enable one to make a much more rigorous testing of theories about relationships between administrative provision, clinical policies and demographic surroundings.

What cannot be escaped, whether comparisons are within or between districts, is the need to agree upon what is comparable with what, and which standards, norms or value judgements we would wish to apply to the information gathered. Comparisons are often considered odious; to help overcome defensive hostility it is desirable to seek prior agreement for such work and reach agreement as to which comparisons can be made.

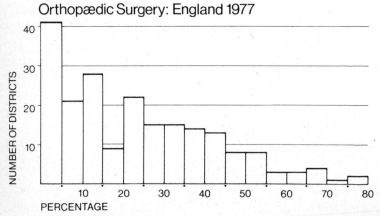

Percentage of Non-urgent Cases Waiting Over One Year: by District:
Orthopædic Surgery: England 1977

Fig. 19    Source: SBH 203

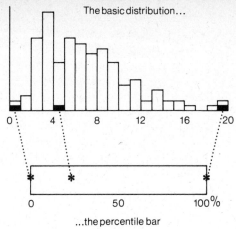

Fig. 20

## Specific Investigations

The comparative investigations outlined above can give some guidance about the relative *amount* of bed stock and the level of *spare capacity* within that bed stock, but they cannot be used with any assurance to study the *use* of beds. The remainder of this chapter outlines some of the work undertaken by various authors attempting to look specifically at problems relating to the three issues of amount of bed stock, the spare capacity required, and the use of hospital beds.

### Assessing the amount of provision required

I have discussed (pp, 6–22) the problems encountered and methods used by those who attempt to determine the need for, and provison of, hospital beds. This book is concerned with the operational management of hospitals rather than the planning of hospitals and, in this context, assessment of required provision can be limited to a comparison of actual bed stock with the planning norms currently in use. This type of crude comparison needs adjustment to take into account the catchment areas of individual specialties. Methods of undertaking this work are discussed by Bennett,[16] West,[142] and Ashford.[6] Comparisons with national or regional norms can, however, be of only limited value because of the value judgements inherent in the setting of norms and the variations of case mix, age, sex and social conditions of the population and the type of hospital accommodation available.

Fig. 21
1977 trauma and orthopaedics speciality profile
(for 202 English Health Districts)

| Indicator | Range | Value for East Sampleshire | Position relative to other districts (expressed as a percentile) |
|---|---|---|---|
| *Descriptive* | | | |
| Balance of Cross Boundary Flow[1] | 0.0%–325.8% | 82.6 | |
| % Residents over 65 | 9.1 – 26.2 | 12.3 | |
| *Demand* | | | |
| Waiting List per Population[2] | 0.0 – 8.9 | 5.5 | |
| % Non-Urgent Cases Waiting over 1 yr | 0.0 – 80.0 | 58.2 | |
| *Input* | | | |
| Beds per Population[2] | 0.1 – 1.0 | 0.35 | |
| Outpatient Sessions per Population[2] | 0.9 – 10.5 | 2.6 | |
| *Process* | | | |
| Length of Stay (days) | 6.5 – 24.4 | 20.3 | |
| Turnover Interval (days) | 0.0 – 13.2 | 3.1 | |
| Day Cases as % of all Inpatients | 0.0 – 51.5 | 37.8 | |
| Total Attendances per New Outpatient | 2.0 – 15.5 | 4.6 | |
| Total Attendances per Clinic | 13.0 – 81.0 | 45.0 | |

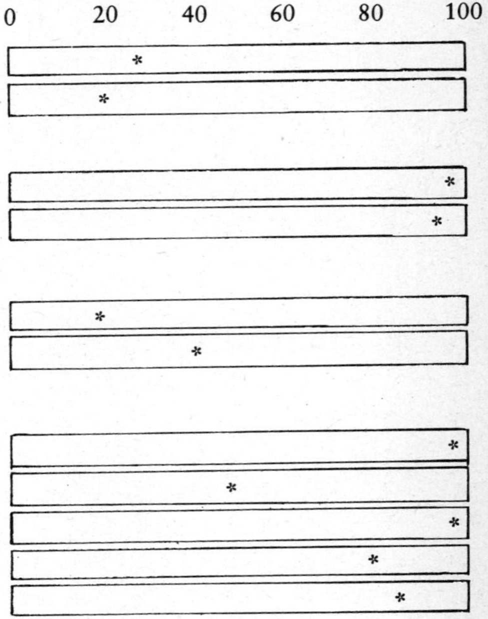

### Assessing the amount of spare capacity required

The amount of spare capacity required depends on the amount of provision available and the variations in admission rates and length of stay patterns of incoming patients. Crude estimates which ignore variations can be made using SH3 data but, of course, can provide only very rough guidelines. Crude assessments can be obtained by making comparisons with units, specialties or hospitals with similar throughputs. An alternative is to make a value judgement about an acceptable turnover interval and relate that to the existing mean length of stay. On a Barber–Johnson diagram one can then read off the percentage emptiness or occupancy and the number of discharges and deaths per bed. This latter figure can be related to the size of the unit and a comparison made between the number of discharges that have been estimated as compared with actual performance in previous years or other units. This type of calculation is illustrated in the work of King and Leach.[82]

More satisfactory assessments require a study of variables not measured by SH3 statistics. The variation of emergency admissions and the hospital's inability to control that variation are of prime interest. Newell,[113] Pike *et al.*[118] and Bithell[18] all suggest that the Poisson distribution provides an adequate statistical description of the arrival of non-waiting-list patients.

### Examining bed use

Table 6 provides a summary of some of the papers that have attempted to analyse the actual use of hospital beds. It attempts to classify methods of examining the three features of bed use referred to earlier – admission, length of stay, and location – in a manner which enables the reader to choose a study most appropriate to his interest. Studies are usually on a current or retrospective basis and in each case one can examine the policy intended or the practice executed. Comparisons can be made of policies against policies, practice against practice, or practice against policies. There are virtually no absolute standards and readers who choose to undertake such investigations are encouraged to review some of the many studies undertaken in order to take advantage of the lessons learned about methodology and then to set their own standards before carrying out their own local investigations. Neither the methods outlined in Table 6 nor any other methods can provide an estimate of inappropriate use unless the participants are prepared to set some standard. Once a standard has been set, then an estimate of the type, cause, and amount of inappropriate use can be obtained.

Table 6
Methods of analysing bed use

| | Area Subject { Practice, Policy | | | Subject | | | Analysis | | | Reviewer | Method and Scope |
|---|---|---|---|---|---|---|---|---|---|---|---|
| | Policy | Practice | Admission | Length of stay | Location | Cross Sectional | Longitudinal | Retrospective | | |
| Chant et al., 1975[29] | | ✓ | | | ✓ | ✓ | | | Independent senior registrars | Random visits incorporating discussion with nurses. Medicine and surgery in two hospitals. |
| Donaldson et al., 1977[46] | | ✓ | | | ✓ | ✓ | | | Nursing staff concerned | Questionnaire to staff, hospitals, residential homes and domiciliary care services of 350 000 population. |
| Fernow et al., 1978[52] | | ✓ | | ✓ | | | | ✓ | Independent clinicians | Data abstracted from case notes. 4 diagnoses, 3 hospitals in two years. |
| Gilkes and Handa, 1974[60] | ✓ | ✓ | | ✓ | | | | ✓ | Consultants | Questionnaire to colleagues. National for 9 operations in ophthalmology. |
| Heasman, 1964[69] | | ✓ | | ✓ | | | | ✓ | Medical researcher | Extracted from HIPE for 1 year for whole of England for two conditions. |
| Heasman & Carstairs, 1971[70] | | ✓ | | ✓ | | | | ✓ | Medical researchers | Extracted from SCRIPS for 1 year – most of Scotland for a number of diagnoses. |
| Hunter, 1972[77] | | ✓ | | ✓ | | | ✓ | | Researcher | Daily study of 198 surgical patients in 3 hospitals. |

| Study | | | | | | | Assessed by | Method |
|---|---|---|---|---|---|---|---|---|
| Lawson, 1974[85] | | | ✓ | ✓ | ✓ | | Consultant | One-day review of 358 patients and of 204 subsequent admissions in one hospital. |
| Logan et al., 1972[88] | ✓ | ✓ | ✓ | ✓ | ✓ | | Medical researchers | Questionnaire to clinicians of 2 specialties in 1 region – results compared with locally collected HAA. |
| Loudon, 1970[90] | | ✓ | ✓ | ✓ | ✓ | | General practitioner | Review/visit of 602 medical and surgical patients in 1 hospital. |
| McArdle et al., 1975[93] | | | | ✓ | ✓ | | Clinicians concerned | Weekly survey over 9 months of 1 female medical ward. |
| Meredith et al., 1968[104] | | ✓ | ✓ | ✓ | ✓ | | Multidisciplinary team | Visit to wards covering 4350 beds in 170 hospitals in Scotland. |
| Murphy, 1977[111] | | | ✓ | ✓ | ✓ | | Medical researchers | Visit/discussion regarding 325 surgical and orthopaedic beds in 4 hospitals. |
| Rubin and Davies, 1975[126] | | | ✓ | ✓ | ✓ | | Researchers | Visit/discussion regarding 1010 patients of 60+ and at least 4 weeks stay in 3 hospitals. |
| Strang et al., 1977[135] | | | ✓ | ✓ | ✓ | | Clinicians and nurses concerned | Questionnaires regarding 1663 surgical, orthopaedic and urological patients. |
| West and Carey, 1978[142] | ✓ | ✓ | | | ✓ | ✓ | Medical researchers | 5038 appendicitis cases extracted from HAA data. |
| Wynne and Hull, 1977[148] | | | | | ✓ | ✓ | Clinicians concerned | 399 emergency paediatric admissions assessed by researcher. |

# 6

# *What can be done to relieve these problems?*

## AVAILABLE TREATMENT

When a doctor has made a diagnosis, he then has to choose what action to take and his options can include a large number of medicines and sometimes operative procedures. Many of these have well-proven efficacy, although the use of randomised controlled trials to ascertain efficacy and effectiveness is a fairly recent development. On the other hand, many treatments have undesirable side-effects and there are also large areas where the benefits of treatment are in doubt. In management, inadequate knowledge of 'disease' processes and their causes leads to ineffective 'treatment' and unexpected side effects. Randomised controlled trials of management activity are virtually unknown.

This chapter provides a framework which lists some of the types of action available and discusses and reviews what is known about their value and side-effects.

---

Chapter 2 demonstrated that many factors influence the allocation and use of hospital beds. Included among these factors are changes in public demand and alterations in the scope and amount of primary care and social services. A consultant's ability to control or influence such issues is extremely limited, so what are the practical steps he can take within the hospital environment to improve the use of hospital beds? I would suggest that there are five areas of interest to the consultant in which he can seek to make changes:

1. The type of bed provision.
2. Administrative policies.
3. Methods of liaison with primary care and social services.
4. The amount of bed provision.
5. Clinical policies.

The following pages set out some of the work which has attempted to improve the use of hospital beds. It is important to understand that, valuable as much of this work is, it is rather like a list of proprietary drugs; each is highly recommended by the maker but shows little evidence of being subject to rigorous test, let alone a randomised controlled trial. This does not mean that the work referred to is of no value, for much of it appears very successful. I would illustrate this by referring to an excellent booklet entitled *Admission of Patients to Hospital*[10] which was published in 1973. Much of the advice in the book is based on the responses to a questionnaire circulated to all large district general hospitals in Great Britain, yet some of the methods and systems proudly displayed by some of those hospitals no longer work. This may be because the method was poor, the application of the method has failed, or some other factor. All the methods may have had some efficacy but not all are effective now.

## The Type of Bed Provision

Traditionally the majority of hospital ward units have catered for all the possible types of admission that can be expected within one specialty. The choice of single specialty wards has meant the concentration of specialised nursing and medical care with its attendant advantages for staff training and organisational convenience and the benefits for the patient of the concentration of such expertise. Variations from this traditional form of organising provision occur when: (a) specialty bed requirements do not fit neatly into multiples of 30 beds (the usual size for a ward unit), thus leading to shared wards; (b) the specialised needs of certain patient groups have to be met by a multi-specialty unit (e.g. intensive therapy units, recovery wards).

The use of progressive patient care methods is discussed at length by Hicks,[72] and Friend[35] shows the effect upon a medical division of instituting ward management with three different levels of care. High quality medical and nursing care and high intensity use of hospital beds are not necessarily incompatible. Some of the variations from the traditional pattern of bed provision have advantages for both individual patient care and the improved use of resources.

## Five-day wards

The twenty-four-hour, seven-day-week nature of hospital emergency departments has typified the public view of all hospital activity. The rest of society works at an entirely different level of activity during the week as compared with the weekends and this is now reflected in hospital activity. This change of attitude and activity combined with the increased number of short-stay admissions now makes it possible for hospitals to run five-day wards. They are normally staffed from Monday mornings to Friday afternoons and are designed to take cases whose length of stay is scheduled to be between one and five days. The established units are more commonly in the surgical specialties. The principle of a five-day ward is to recognise the trough in bed occupancy which occurs in all general hospitals at weekends and lower the overall staffing level accordingly. This reduces the number of available bed days – but these are usually bed days which are totally wasted. Considerable revenue saving is made by not staffing the ward for two whole days and three nights. Certain revenue savings also accrue in other (non-nurse) staffing areas and in expenditure other than on salaries. Such units are helpful in providing a different type of nurse manning pattern. This is claimed to help nurse recruitment, retention of staff, and staff morale. Five-day wards are reported to be liked by patients and it is also claimed that the discipline imposed on patient scheduling discourages wasted bed days. Discussions of five-day wards may be found in the *British Medical Journal*,[21] Ingram and Traynor,[79] Clayton *et al.*,[31] and Towers.[138]

The disadvantages of five-day wards seem to lie primarily in the difficulty of avoiding a tail-off of activity towards the end of the week if one- and two-day stay patients cannot be scheduled for operation or treatment on Thursdays and Fridays. Other difficulties can arise in transferring cases not fit for discharge on the Friday afternoon. Certain criticisms have also been offered regarding lack of nursing continuity and stimulus and the creation of 'heavier' nursing on other units which no longer have a balanced workload.

## Programmed investigation units

A programmed investigation unit was first described by Longson and Young,[89] as 'an in-patient department providing facilities for all tests used in medicine.' It provides basic minimum nursing care and is suitable for ambulant patients who can care for themselves. Longson's original paper and a subsequent DHSS publication[41] describe seven years' experience of operating such a unit at Manchester Royal

Infirmary. The unit operates on a five-day basis and was established on the assumptions that (a) the 'first generation' of investigations could be predicted after the initial out-patient consultation and screening procedures; (b) in most cases the 'first generation' of investigations would include all the major procedures required in a particular case ('second generation' tests, which derive from the first would be simple to organise, for example, venepunctures); and (c) hospital doctors would modify their pattern of work in out-patient clinics to describe more accurately the purpose of admission and to predict the relevant investigations. Within the unit, beds are not allocated to individual clinicians but the admitting clinician retains full clinical responsibility for the patient. The organisation of the sequence of the tests and the date of admission are both the responsibility of the unit and are incorporated into a timetable agreed with the investigative departments. The value of such a unit lies in its ability to time admission to suit the convenience of the patient, to arrange tests in a clinically compatible sequence, and to increase efficiency by avoiding unnecessary delays which commonly lead to inappropriate length of in-patient stay. The separation of investigatory work from the preponderance of work caused by emergency admissions to general medical wards enables admissions to be made with greater certainty and investigations to be carried out with greater logic and expertise under less pressure and with less waste of bed days. The Manchester unit has also been able to reduce waiting lists and waiting times for patients requiring in-patient investigations.

To date, few criticisms of planned investigation units have been forthcoming. Longson[89] states that the existence of a unit means that ward rounds and medical cover have to be extended to an additional ward, but the advantages appear to outweigh the small inconvenience. Longson also claims that very little deflection of out-patient investigation has been made to the unit and any fear of overinvestigation is completely refuted, in that careful programming appears to lessen investigations as compared with previous haphazard investigational patterns. Gandy's[57] evaluation of the unit concluded that the introduction of planned investigation units 'is likely to have a beneficial effect on the use of medical beds in any major hospital and, in turn, on the patients treated there.' The establishment of further programmed investigation units has not been speedy, although some twenty units of various sizes are known to exist (e.g. Newcastle Victoria Infirmary, Sachdev *et al.*[129]) A possible reason for the slow take-up may lie in the variation of suitable workload between units. Davies[37] quotes proportions to range from under 10% to 32%, with the larger proportions being in teaching and research hospitals. There are however, examples of small programmed investigation units working in non-teaching hospitals and Davies has outlined the alternative of a planned investigation bed on a general medical ward (see also DHSS[40]). Whilst this suggestion does not have all the benefits of a separate unit it appears to have two additional advantages; weekend use of the bed can be made, and the improved efficiency of the running of this single bed can be 'catching' and help to improve the management of the rest of the ward.

**Admission wards**
A further alternative to the traditional ward pattern is to separate some group of admissions during the early part of their stay. Types of admission wards include emergency admission units and pre-operative planned admission units.

Emergency admission units are designed to separate either minor cases or more disruptive cases from the main wards. Examples include the provision of a special unit for admissions during the night and a unit which is staffed twenty-four hours a day to take short-stay (i.e. up to three days) cases. The fluctuation of admission to such units can be described mathematically.[118] The value of such units lies in their ability to shield other wards from disruptive admissions, which aids the planning of main ward admissions and work. Disruption is of two kinds; firstly, the noise and disruption of admitting a late night patient and, secondly, the disruption to cold admission scheduling caused by short-stay emergencies. The disadvantages lie in the tendency to disperse staffing skills in dealing with emergencies to at least two sites and to cause a concentration of heavy nursing on the main wards.

A pre-operative planned admission unit is described by Duthie *et al*.[48] Pre-operative patients are admitted to, and investigated in, a special ward which consists of hotel-type accommodation and has minimal nursing care. The patients meet the staff who will care for them after operation but do not go to the main ward until after their operation. Advantages include gradual acclimatisation of patients to the hospital environment, concentration of pre-operative examination and investigation skills, identification of one point for patient admission, avoiding the scattering and 'loss' of patients, a contribution to lower infection rates, and a reduction in pre- and postoperative stay. The main disadvantages cited are the change in environment, – surroundings and people – for the patient, and the inevitable lack of continuity of nursing care.

Admission ward units in multispecialty situations are most frequently criticised because of the difficulty of providing the admission unit with all the different types of skills required and also the tendency to deplete the main wards of those very same skills.

### Predischarge wards

The criticisms made of multispecialty admission wards can in theory be surmounted by using a predischarge ward. Transferring patients to such a ward towards the end of their stay means that intensive nursing care of a specialist nature is not required on that ward. The establishment of a predischarge unit involves setting up a separate ward unit with a relatively low level of nurse staffing, able to take predischarge cases from many specialties and, preferably, patients of both sexes. The principle is that it becomes the buffer ward which responds to the fluctuations of emergency admissions, (but at the other end of the patient's stay) and that the ward is used for short-stay (i.e. up to seven days) patients whose bed is required on the main ward in order to accommodate emergency admissions or more seriously ill patients. The concept is frequently applied by using outlying hospital units, but its incorporation into a district general hospital has been described by Zinovieff *et al.*[152] Its value from the patient's point of view is that it provides a quieter and more restful environment. For the hospital, it provides a safety valve for ward pressure and can contribute to overall patient throughput. The disadvantage, for both patients and nurses, is the lack of continuity of care. Such a unit also contributes to making nursing on the main ward more continuously heavy. The lack of published evidence of similar experiments is seen by some to indicate that the disadvantages outweigh the benefits, particularly with the steady fall in length of stay in the surgical specialties which are most suitable for the use of the predischarge ward. On the other hand, the use of predischarge methods may in fact be so commonly practised by using peripheral units (convalescent or preconvalescent hospitals) that publication of results is not undertaken. (A review of preconvalescent hospitals was published by Hughes and Miller[76]).

### Combining alternatives

Some of the more common alternatives to the traditional ward arrangement have been listed above. Some can be combined and two such arrangements are the mixing of elective surgery and programmed investigation in a five-day ward, and the use of a five-day ward unit at night as an emergency admission unit. The former is described by

Burgess *et al.*[22] and examples of the latter are to be found at Northwick Park Hospital, London, and North Tees General Hospital, Stockton on Tees.

## Administrative Policies

The way in which a consultant organises his firm and a hospital manages its affairs can clearly contribute to or detract from the efficient use of hospital beds. All hospitals admit and discharge patients, but the way these activities are carried out, the policies used, and the degree of formalisation of these policies vary considerably. Although it is difficult to isolate the precise contribution of these supporting functions, attention to some of the following policies can make a contribution to the effective use of beds.

### The establishment of information systems
Admission decisions are rarely made in the absence of any information, but many argue that more effective decisions can be made by having accurate and timely information readily available for the consultant and other staff who make decisions on the admission of patients. Information systems which provide data about current bed states, outstanding waiting-list cases, and previous admission patterns are sometimes concentrated in one location or under the control of one member of staff. These information systems exist at ward or unit level (e.g. Sutton,[136] Hicks[72]), at divisional level (e.g. Murray and Topley[112]), or at hospital level (e.g. Chubb and Hodgkinson[30]). A useful review of information rooms is provided by Griffiths.[62 63]

Information systems are rather like clothes – they are best tailored for the individual's taste and will be changed as fashion changes. In no way can they be considered unnecessary in our climate!

### Scheduling and control

#### 1. Emergency admissions
Having established information flows, then a controlling mechanism is required. Bed bureaux are commonly used to undertake this function (e.g. Grant,[61] Marshall and Spencer,[98] on a city basis, or Hicks,[72] on a unit basis). Such units can make best use of beds by a full understanding of theory (e.g. Newell,[113] Pike[118]) and local experience of emergency admission patterns.

## 2. Planned admission

The calling of planned admissions must be related, at a minimum, to emergency admission patterns and occupancy levels. As notice is required for the patients, this means that the hospital has to make some prediction about future levels of occupancy and likely emergency admissions and discharges of all types. In situations of low bed emptiness this requires a fine balance to be made between the amount of notice given to the patient and the degree of certainty that can be attached to having an available bed. In general, the longer the notice the less the certainty and vice versa. The prediction of discharge dates has received the attention of doctors, administrators, nurses and mathematicians,[19 28] but so far has not proved to be a well-refined art.

The scheduling of admissions based on past performance (without any attempt to refine discharge prediction) appears to be a solid base on which to build admission patterns. The analysis of existing emergency and cold admission patterns, and the simulation of possible changes in policy, can be used to identify desirable changes[109] and improve performance.[39]

Two further problems in calling planned admission cases are failure of patients to attend when called and patients not being fit for operation when called. The avoidance of short call notice, the regular review of waiting lists, and the maintenance of short-call registers can contribute to the reduction of attendance failures.[39 150] Pre-admission clinics (quite apart from any clinical advantages) are a method of eliminating the calling of patients not fit for operation.[23 35] One important value of pre-admission clinics lies in their ability to save on pre-operative bed occupancy. Most hospitals call a patient for admission after the patient has spent a period of time on the waiting list, but a number of units are attempting to give the patient a booked date for admission on attendance at the out-patient department. An example of this policy is published by Southam and Talbot.[133]

## The pooling of beds

Coping with the fluctuating demand for admission and bed days is easier in a large unit than in a series of small ones. The mathematical theory of pooling beds is straightforward. An Oxford Regional Hospital Board pamphlet[115] demonstrates that 'given random demand, 100 beds used jointly compared with 10 separate units each of 10 beds increases potential bed-days by over 10% and at the same time considerably reduces the number of days when extra beds are required.' A considerable amount of theoretical work has been undertaken on this subject, particularly in comparing four 30-bedded ward units with 120-bed units in the designing of new district general hospitals.[72 91] In practice, pooling of beds is done in a number of ways, which may be by pooling all the beds in one specialty, all beds in like specialties, all acute beds in a hospital, or all acute beds in a district. The value of pooling lies in the ability to admit extra cases within the same number of beds and at the same time reduce the frequency of erecting extra beds or turning patients away. The principal disadvantage is simply that patients previously kept together stand a greater chance of being scattered between a larger number of locations. This makes for nursing difficulties when patients of different specialties are on the same ward and also requires the medical team to hunt more widely for its patients on a ward round and cover a greater distance when on emergency call. In practice the points for and against have been difficult to evaluate and Hicks points out that the theory and simulation models he described have 'not been tested or validated in use.' Some of the difficulty of testing the theory lies in the fact that bed pooling in an informal way is normal hospital activity, particularly when under pressure. Marshall and Spencer[98] show that, when pooling was introduced in a district general hospital, a marked increase in patient throughput was observed but 'this increased efficiency in numerical terms was not mirrored by an improvement in the morale of the doctors and nurses working on the wards, who were subjected to new pressures and considered that at times the standard of patient care deteriorated.' This comment should perhaps be taken in the context of the severe nurse staffing shortage at the hospital concerned. The work appears to validate the theory even though its application may not have been appropriate in the particular circumstances.

### Overall scheduling of ward and support department activity

This book concentrates on the 'bed' as an important resource. Its use depends very much on the availability of many support services. The day-to-day scheduling of these activities has been aided by modelling. This work has been particularly prevalent in surgical specialties, where the theatre is a crucial part of the total activity. The work of operational research specialists predominates in this field.[74 92 140 146]

Some of the difficulties of the scheduling approach lie in the need to collect large volumes of information on a continuous basis and to have somewhat complex mathematical manipulations of the information gathered. In such circumstances the understanding of the system by its users is of key importance and it has not always proved possible to transfer such knowledge and commitment from year to year during the inevitable changes of staff.

## Liaison with Social Services and Primary Care

The blocking of acute hospital beds by patients who could more appropriately be cared for at home or in long-stay hospital accommodation is a problem more easily quantified than resolved. Close cooperation with social work and primary care staff has been claimed to be of significant importance in improving bed blocking and patient turnover,[13 14] although I have been unable to find much published evidence on this subject.

## The Amount of Bed Provision

The treatments described so far are 'medical' in flavour, but 'surgical' techniques are also available. Bed allocation can be reduced or increased. Reduction of bed complement should be preceded by a search for alternative use and any closure should be accompanied by a reallocation of the financial saving made. Calls for extra provision should be considered in three stages: (1) Is there any vacant staffed accommodation that could be made available? (2) Is there any vacant unstaffed accommodation (e.g. closed wards) that may require upgrading? (3) Can other hospitals or districts provide the service at a satisfactory level? Unless new accommodation is planned to replace that which is outdated, these questions should be considered before additional building is started. Simulation techniques can be used to examine alternatives.[143]

The strengths of this type of action lie in the fact that the need for capital development is minimised and even dispensed with. There is a tendency to get better value for money in that more cases are treated (if you are prepared to assume outcome is effective); reallocation is more speedy than capital development; finally, this crude review method does not require some of the more costly and elaborate information systems needed for other methods of improving resource use. There are three main weaknesses: total expenditure tends to increase when throughput increases (even though unit cost per case may fall); reallocation means bargaining with 'bed landlords' and frequently such bargaining is the cause of animosity and staff unrest; changes in fabric need additional small capital or revenue expenditure which some organisations have difficulty in providing. A case study describing this type of action appears in a paper by King *et al.*[83]

## Clinical Policies

The four previous sections have attempted to outline some of the methods available to help improve the use of hospital beds, with discussion of the advantages and disadvantages of the methods outlined. Such a format is not appropriate for this section because, as an administrator, I am unable to judge the effectiveness of some of the aspects of clinical policies. However, changes in clinical policy frequently have significant implications for the use of resources. To the clinician who is primarily concerned with the effect of that policy on an invididual patient, the implications of his decisions upon resources seem to him at least secondary if not irrelevant. In this section I would like to discuss three issues; first, some of the evidence that indicates how clinical decisions affect resource use; second, the doubts that exist about doctors' attitudes to such issues; and third, the suggestion that the 'side-effect' of resource use should be considered along with other side-effects when examining existing and new clinical policies.

### Clinical policies and resource implications

Decisions made about the necessity for admission, the length of stay of the patient, and the location of patients all influence resource use. Let us look at some illustrations. The advantages of admission for a proportion of acute myocardial infarction cases has been questioned,[73][101][102] and the subject is the source of much debate (e.g. Royal College of Physicians Working Party[123]). Any change in policy in a diagnostic category like acute myocardial infarction, which is both a common cause of admission and a high user of bed days, will significantly alter overall bed provision requirements. The same diagnostic group can be used to illustrate the impact of policies regarding length of stay.[59][66][78] Considerable variations in length of stay pattern can be observed in most specialties for many conditions and, in the absence of clinical evidence as to the value of longer stay, it is not surprising if the clinician is pressed by those who are concerned with resource provision to reconsider his policy. Such pressure is only strengthened by published examples of the re-examination of length of stay policies.[47][132] Advances in clinical practice and pharmacology can completely alter the pattern of medicine or surgery practised in a ward and thus the requirement for beds. A startling example of this is the introduction of metronidazole in the management of appendicectomy. Formerly, emergency appendicectomy was associated with a high incidence of abscess formation and consequently the patients remained in hospital for a protracted period. Metronidazole has changed all this and, in a recent experimental study[145], the incidence of abscess formation following emergency appendicectomy was substantially and significantly reduced.

Clinical decisions about the location of patients (i.e. choosing the type of accommodation) are probably influenced by the type of accommodation available, but the amount of misplacement suggested by some authors[29 112] indicates that clinical decisions must take at least some of the responsibility for misuse of beds. Highly expensive facilities utilised by patients not requiring such resources must either deny those resources to other more needful patients or expend money that could be more efficiently used in providing a different level of support. The question of inappropriate location is two-sided. Is it the wrong type of accommodation or has the wrong patient been selected? The subject is debated by Martindale and Garfield[99] in discussing the use of neurosurgical beds and neuroradiological facilities by certain groups of patients at the expense of more needy groups. The debate about the impact of clinical policy on bed use is not simply a question of using or not using a bed. The economist describes 'cost' as including 'benefits forgone'. In other words, utilisation of a scarce resource by a patient who can receive little benefit from admission to an acute hospital bed can mean that the admission of other patients who might benefit more from such a facility is delayed or even forgone.

## The clinician's attitude to resource implications

In examining attitudes, I would like to concentrate on the actions of clinicians rather than the views they express. The types of policy variation outlined above raise at least two issues. First, there appears to be a considerable time-lag in the take-up of new clinical policies and, second, the resource implication of any change appears to be a minor if not forgotten aspect.

The question of time-scales is illustrated when examining day-case surgery. Day-case operations were first reported in the *British Medical Journal* in 1909,[114] but the beginnings of day surgery are more correctly dated to 1955.[51] By the 1960s, day surgery was hardly common practice and even today, despite a stream of papers pointing to the clinical acceptibility of day-case and out-patient surgery, the practice (though widespread) is by no means uniformly undertaken. A helpful review of some literature was provided by Boardman and Griffiths[20] in a paper which goes on to describe out-patient surgery in orthopaedics. Further references can be found for general surgery,[417 128]

gynaecology,[33 139] and ophthalmology.[65] The time-lag in the accept-
ance of new policies is not merely a medical problem but one with
resource implications.

A second criticism of the clinician's attitude lies in the apparent lack
of concern with resource implications when examining a new treatment. The introduction of cimetidine has been accompanied by well
over 500 papers in medical and pharmaceutical journals. A few papers
make cursory reference to the effect on bed use, but not one paper has
addressed the matter in a manner which compares with the rigour
adopted in the randomised controlled trials of the clinical outcome.

### Resource implications – an important side effect

In this section, I am not trying to suggest that resource implications
should be paramount over all other issues when examining a change of
policy, nor am I requesting clinicians to review policies with the sole
purpose of improving the use of hospital beds. I would ask that clinicians examine all the side effects of existing and changed clinical
policies. Any change which saves resources can contribute to improving the care and treatment of other patients, although in some cases it
must be recognised that additional or alternative resources have to be
expended before a resource saving is attained in terms of beds. Policies
such as appropriate length of stay can too easily fall into a pattern
which is of unproven validity. The need to test clinical criteria is not
always an accepted challenge within the medical profession. Re-
examination of traditional patterns can lead not only to improved use
of hospital resources but also to improved clinical results.

## Relating Techniques to Problems

Chapter 5 outlined investigatory methods which might contribute to
diagnosing problems of the amount, use and spare capacity of bed provision. The solution of these problems might require an increase or
decrease in the amount of provision, increase or decrease of the
amount of spare capacity, or a more appropriate use of beds. The
methods listed in this chapter are not, of course, appropriate to all of
these problems although some of the actions outlined can aid more
than one problem. Table 7 is prepared as a crude guide to linking the
action required to the problem diagnosed.

All these methods are subject to the overriding question of how such
changes can be made or encouraged. This crucial subject is examined in
the next chapter.

*Table 7*
**Bed use: relating available methods to problems presented**

| Methods available | Inadequate bed stock | Too much bed stock | Inadequate spare capacity | Too much spare capacity | Inappropriate use |
|---|---|---|---|---|---|
| **Type of bed provision** | | | | | |
| Progressive patient care | ? | × | ? | × | ? |
| Five-day wards | ? | √ | × | √ | ? |
| Programmed investigation units | ? | × | × | × | √ |
| Admission wards | √ | × | √ | × | ? |
| Predischarge wards | √ | × | √ | × | ? |
| **Clinical policies** | | | | | |
| Home care not admission | √ | × | √ | × | √ |
| Out-patient not in-patient | √ | × | √ | × | √ |
| Reduction in length of stay | √ | × | √ | × | √ |
| **Administrative policies** | | | | | |
| Establishment of information systems | ? | ? | ? | ? | ? |
| Scheduling and control of admissions | √ | × | √ | ? | × |
| Discharge prediction | ? | × | ? | × | × |
| Pooling of beds | √ | × | √ | × | × |
| Waiting list management | ? | × | × | √ | × |
| Overall scheduling | ? | × | ? | ? | × |
| Liaison with social services and primary care | √ | × | ? | × | √ |
| Adjusting amount of provision | √ | √ | √ | √ | ? |

KEY  √ Highly likely to help
? May help
× Will not help

# 7

# *How can change be achieved?*

## CLINICAL PRACTICE

The natural outcome of many diseases is spontaneous resolution without any medical intervention, but there are vast areas where intervention is required. Whilst the sum total of knowledge in medicine is formidable and the application of that knowledge impressive, there are still diseases which remain incurable. For the individual practitioner there are many problems. He cannot gain and apply all the available knowledge, he cannot guarantee that all patients will comply with his advice, and he finds that much of his practice is in the areas of uncertainty where apparently efficacious intervention sometimes fails and where the placebo effect is encountered. Medicine is not merely a science, partly because scientific knowledge is incomplete and more importantly because the application of medicine to each individual patient is specific and personal.

In management, the sum total of knowledge is not so impressive. Many problem areas do not appear to be amenable to correction, individual managers fail to obtain and apply the knowledge available, organisations fail to respond to advice offered, even when correct, and on other occasions improvements occur without apparent corrective action being taken.

This chapter makes observations about the relationship between information, decisions, actions, and results. It begins by showing the frailty of quantitative measurement, well-designed systems, and good practice, in the light of human attitudes and behaviour. It concludes with advice aimed at minimising the frustrations and maximising the success for those seeking to achieve a better use of hospital beds.

This book, in attempting to provide an analytical framework, may seem to suggest a straightforward relationship between identifying a problem, choosing a corrective remedy, and achieving successful change. If that is the case, this chapter is designed to shatter that illusion. Producing change in an organisation like the health service is an awesome task. The newly-appointed physician who is allocated only six general medical beds and then spends five years engineering a larger allocation may be forgiven for feeling that the organisation has some personal grudge against him. Time after time, clinicians, nurses and administrators feel frustrated in their efforts to make better use of resources.

CASE STUDY
A medical division was presented with information relating to the uneven distribution of workload between five medical wards. The information presented satisfied the majority of the criteria suggested in Chapter 4, i.e., accuracy, completeness, understandability, timeliness, appropriate quantity and orginality. The uneven flow of admissions (illustrated in Fig. 22) was perceived as a problem by the nursing, junior

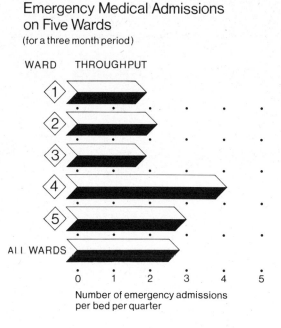

**Emergency Medical Admissions on Five Wards**
(for a three month period)

Number of emergency admissions per bed per quarter

Fig. 22

medical and administrative staff. The situation was exacerbated for them by the fact that the wards with the highest number of emergency admissions also had a higher number of 'cold' admissions. The division, however, did not see a problem. To them, the information was not relevant and no action was taken.

A similar problem of uneven distribution, this time between hospitals (see Fig. 23), was presented to a division in an identical manner. The result was agreement by the division that the information and the problem were relevant. Action was subsequently taken to adjust junior medical staffing in order to alleviate the difficulties encountered.

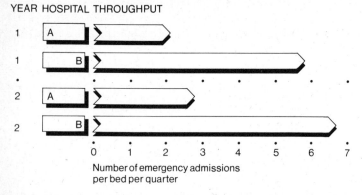

### Emergency Medical Admissions to Two Hospitals
(comparing the first three months of two successive years)

Fig. 23

Different responses to similar information about similar problems are not uncommon. These two events, however, appear in particularly stark contrast because they were consecutive items at one meeting of one division. A keen sportsman present at that meeting would have detected that the first item was played as a 'friendly', but the second had the determination, excitement and tension of a cup-tie. The comments of the individual clinicians after the meeting ranged from attempted rational explanations for seemingly inconsistent behaviour, to cynical remarks about the balance of voters between hospitals on the night concerned. In circumstances like this, there is often more at stake than information about comparative workloads and we must accept that information of itself cannot ensure action – especially when it collides with prejudice. Information which hints at change can be threatening and, inevitably, 'attitudes are resistent to change; that is their function'.[75]

Many hospital consultants find that it is becoming increasingly difficult to develop their specialty for the benefit of their patients. Merely identifying and expressing a need no longer guarantees that resources will be provided to meet that need. Perhaps this was never in fact the case, but today's consultants find that less credence than ever appears to be given to their clinical training, status and intellectual ability when they make a case to a financially embarrassed health service for additional resources. The changing structure of the health service leaves some consultants with the feeling that not only are the rules constantly being changed, but also that the game is always played away from home. Administrators, on the other hand, suggest that many consultants have an unrealistic approach to the financial constraints that are imposed upon the health service. Clinicians and administrators look at each other's attitudes and (with some justification) each side feels that there are none so blind as those who will not see.

## The Inertia of Organisations

It is easier to quote examples of resistance to rational arguments which suggest change than it is to explain why such resistance is encountered. However, if we consider a sufficiently large group of case studies we may begin to understand more about behaviour within an organisation and develop a range of strategies which we can call upon to try to combat resistance. Achieving change within a large organisation is complicated by the fact that one has to cope not only with the behaviour of individuals, but also with the behaviour of the organisation itself and its constituent parts. The way an organisation works is difficult to understand, not only for outsiders who come into contact with it, but also for those who work within it. Many of us are curious about how and why decisions were made in the past and also how we should act and how the organisation might react in the future. For instance, when seeking additional resources we can refer to past 'form' and then make a case based on certain assumptions about the likely response of the organisation. The formulation and presentation of the case is influenced by our assumptions about how it will be received. Three common assumptions made about decision making in large organisations are:

1. *That an organisation will act like a somewhat rational individual*
Rational man has goals and objectives. In order to meet those goals he generates alternative courses of action. He considers the consequences of each of the alternatives and finally makes choices. He is the classic 'economic' man who chooses the most efficient alternative. Rational behaviour recognises that goals can conflict, but it can resolve such conflicts. This activity includes matching means to ends. It requires 'wants' to be cardinally ranked and may also require a recognition of what is unobtainable. It is a very commendable theory, but does the health service behave like a rational individual? It is often difficult for an organisation as small as an orthopaedic division to act like a rational individual, let alone a health district or a health service.

2. *That an organisation will behave as a ponderous bureaucratic machine*
Within an organisation, decisions are not made in a vacuum which allows precise rational thinking. Decisions result from an interaction between groups and each group unpacks the same problem in a different way. In his book, *Essence of Decision*, Allison[3] suggests that organisations have certain characteristics and he describes (amongst others) the following tendencies.

Organisations: (a) have standard operating procedures (e.g. committee structures);
(b) give sequential attention to problems that arise;
(c) form coalitions rather than resolve conflicts;
(d) avoid uncertainty, and
(e) learn, but slowly.

These characteristics will be familiar to those who work in the NHS and it may come as somewhat of a surprise and even a comfort to know that Allison's book was analysing the decisions of American and Russian governments and their armed forces during the Cuban missile crisis!

3. *That an organisation will respond only to power of personalities and political manoeuvring.*
Another assumption that can be made about organisations is that they are merely a collection of individuals and groups. Personalities and political groups interact to shape and share power. They behave like players in some sort of bargaining game and their choice of issues for discussion tends to be very specific. Some of the characteristics of this political model are:

(a) bargaining takes place either with real issues or through the provision or withholding of information;

(b) that a formal position allows a particular place or role in the game;

(c) individuals and groups tend to be defensive – risk-taking is unusual;

(d) communication tends to be up and down structures rather than across, and

(e) the speed of response is fast.

Once again these characteristics are not unknown in the behaviour of groups within the NHS.

Clearly each of the three assumptions is highly caricatured, but if we apply each model to one simple example – that of an orthopaedic division making a case for additional hospital beds – we may begin to build a framework upon which we can more confidently tackle the task of achieving change in an organisation. For the purposes of simplicity, let us assume that the division concerned is well-staffed, has adequate theatre and out-patient provision, can obtain most of the equipment it needs, but is short of beds.

The division might consider three options, the rational, bureaucratic and political.

## A rational case

Orthopaedic surgeons must recognise that what is obvious to them may not be so obvious to others and, in particular, to managers and other laymen. They should explain that some patients in the community suffer considerable pain because of diseased joints. Orthopaedic surgeons have the technical ability to relieve that pain and also return those patients to an improved life-style which will benefit the whole community. In this instance, the failure to relieve pain is simply due to inadequate resource provision and, in particular, hospital beds. The division's case highlights the unmet need for joint replacement with the figures from the growing waiting list and the evidence gleaned from a survey by the district community physician and a group of local general practitioners on the incidence and prevalence of diseased joints of patients in the district.

Having identified the need, the division then proceeds to demonstrate that it does not have spare capacity to cope with the need, neither is there any opportunity for improving its existing way of working in order to release some spare capacity to cope with the unmet need. The demonstration of good performance is wide-ranging. Bed emptiness is extremely low and bed provision is lower than all norms established at local, regional and national levels. There is little or no bed-blocking, due to excellent cooperation with a well-run geriatric service and cooperative social services. Patient length of stay on the main wards cannot be significantly shortened to save beds. This is supported by comparison with other similar units and regional and national figures, which show the division to have very short length of stay patterns. Day-case theatre capacity is available, but no expansion of use can be undertaken because all cases suitable for day-case care are already being so treated. Much of the work of the division has been subject to randomised controlled trials on matters of clinical outcome, need for admission, and length of stay, and the results of such trials show the division in a very favourable light.

The divison feels the case for making provision for an unmet demand is clear. The wherewithal to meet that demand is not present within the division and so it has to seek for other ways of meeting that demand. The options open to it are few and most of them appear impracticable or costly (in every sense). Prevention of occurrence is not yet proving viable and busing patients to the nearest point of spare capacity proves difficult to arrange. The method of meeting the unmet demand is almost self-selecting – more resources (in this case hospital beds) are required. Having identified the need and selected the best method of meeting that need the division then proceeds to provide more details about the likely outcome of such action and the anticipated cost. The results are predicted in terms of reduced waiting time and consequent suffering, less time away from work, a decrease in waiting numbers, and a better deployment of under-used resources (e.g. theatre staff). In collaboration with appropriate advisers from the works department, rough estimates of new and up-graded premises are obtained. The case when agreed by the division is typed, illustrated and bound and fit for any receiving body.

The receipt of the division's case by a rational organisation might be as follows. The case would be favourably received because it is well presented and logical. Needs and alternatives would be re-examined closely. The chosen strategy of additional beds would be particularly closely examined, firstly by studying the activity of the division itself and then by widening the field of study by examining the allocation and use of beds made by other specialties within the district. As the division accepted the need and then tried to encompass the need within its existing activity, similarly a health district would attempt to meet the need from within the district's resources. It would look for changes in bed allocation and clinical policy which would make staffed beds available at no additional revenue cost. The division's task of selecting its priority (more beds for joint replacement) was in this case very simple, but a district management team's choice of priorities is almost always more complex. The orthopaedic division's case is one of many and, where resources are limited (and they always are), choices between desirable options have to be made. The division's case may be accepted and funded but, alternatively, it may be accepted and yet, because funds are not immediately available, placed on a list of desirable objectives and the consequences of delayed implementation have to be faced.

## A bureaucratic case

The bureaucratic model takes on board as much rationality as it can within the constraints that organisational operation allows. Let us examine five of the constraints which Allison observed and see how the division might need to adapt its case.

1. Like most large organisations, the NHS has many standardised operating procedures. Methods of consultation with staff and the public over the closure of hospitals are an example. More commonly recognised are the formal committee structures and committee time-tables through which a case for additional resources has to pass. An application for the establishment of a senior registrar post can pass through a dozen committees before formal approval is granted and even then funding for the post may not be guaranteed. The orthopaedic division's case will not necessarily pass through medical executive committee, to district management team, and thence to the health authority, but may have to suffer many diversions. The medical executive committee (MEC) may want the advice of the theatre users committee, the district management team (DMT) requires the approval of the district medical committee and the health care planning teams and the district health authority will wish to consult the regional health authority (RHA) on the availability of capital money. A division needs to allow time to chart and steer a course through the complex waters of committee structures.

2. Sequential attention is well favoured in medical committees. The MEC may agree that the orthopaedic surgeons have a very laudable case, but suggest that the surgeons must recognise that as relative new-comers they cannot expect all facilities immediately. The physicians

have spent twenty years building their empire and the surgeons must be patient and await their turn behind the already accepted proposals from the divisions of anaesthetics and cardiology. The sequential attention problem will face the orthopaedic division at every stage. The DMT will also stress the need to repair the boiler house chimney and up-grade the kitchens before any more patient accommodation can be used. The RHA also remind the DMT that accommodation and revenue has been reserved for the regional centre for respiratory physiology, and, as the respiratory physician takes up post next May, the facilities must be prepared immediately. Unless the division has such a strong case that it clearly justifies queue-jumping, the only course of action is to get in quick with its case.

3.  Coalition in preference to conflict occurs throughout most groups within an organisation. Divisions, DMT's and health authorities often prefer at each level to join together in pressing the immediately higher committee for an expansion of the budget in preference to directing its attention to making priority decisions within the budgets provided. If a division wishes to short-circuit a long process, it might consider looking for suitable coalitions at an early stage. Would a joint case with the division of geriatrics avoid some difficulties in making choices and at the same time provide an even stronger case?

4.  Organisations try to avoid uncertainty by such mechanisms as the production of plans and long-term budgets and by seeking to avoid party politics in local policy matters. The strong emphasis on planning means that divisions need to ensure that their ideas are quickly incorporated into the district plan, and thence into the regional planning cycle. If this is not immediately possible, the division should try to demonstrate where their current proposals match or complement the existing plan for the district.

5.  An organisation learns (and changes) through serious performance failures (e.g. Normansfield, Farleigh, and Ely enquiries), budget famine (e.g. the wrong end of RAWP, or by budget feast (an unusual occurrence, but illustrated by the £9 million hand-out for waiting lists). These three learning experiences must be spotted by divisions and used to the full. If a performance failure occurs the event should be turned to the advantage of the division as soon as possible. A serious outbreak of sepsis must first be controlled and then its recurrence avoided, but the latter activity provides a splendid opportunity for the division to

press its point. Turning to budget famine, the division needs to have ideas of where savings can be made (elsewhere in the organisation) in order to point out to the hard-done-by organisation where some resources can come from and, at the same time, ensure that at least part of the saving goes to the division. Finally, the budget feast usually requires speedily available plans for immediate expenditure of money. The division should ensure that at least part of its case can be converted into such a plan at very short notice.

Organisational behaviour clearly alters the rational model that we began with and provides an alternative model on which to base assumptions about how we think an organisation will respond to a case for additional resources. At the same time we have examined how the division might respond to such organisational behaviour and, in so doing we move towards a third option – the political model.

### A political case

Allison[3] outlined five of the characteristics of the political model and whilst there are others available, let us see how those five might affect the orthopaedic division.

1. Discussion between divisions about agreeing a common policy may be wide-ranging, but the real bargaining will be on parochial and very tangible issues. A common policy on the management of heart disease is relatively easily arranged compared with deciding how the divisions of general medicine and cardiology will arrange cover for 'on call' and who will carry the 'bleep'. For the orthopaedic division this means that it will have to bargain mainly on 'crunch' issues, like the management of the Accident and Emergency Department and its junior staffing rather than on more innocuous threats of 'not supporting your case if you don't support mine'.

2. Debating and bargaining hinge partly on ability and personality, but very often rely on formal status and knowledge. When a DMT is discussing nurse training the nursing officer will tend to control the situation but, if the next item on the agenda is 'cash limits', then the finance officer takes over the key position. Similarly, within a division, the views of the nursing and junior staff are noted, but can easily be overridden by the consultant. The implication of this behaviour for the orthopaedic division is that it must understand who holds the formal positions of influence at each stage of the committee structure and see

to it that those individuals are properly briefed and conversant with the case of the division when the formal meeting takes place.

3.  Large scale changes in policy and funding are unusual. Organisations seldom make major changes in direction, but prefer to take small steps, thus not moving far from their existing position. The NHS dislikes major changes and finds it difficult to close hospitals or establish new services quickly. In this climate the division is perhaps wiser if it does not push its luck by going for wholesale change but works instead on the wedge principle. The division should obtain some of its requirements and then argue for the rest later. This can be done by declaring the sequence or, less honestly, by arranging for the first step to force the provision of the second (e.g. 'We've got the staff but they cannot work without the equipment and we do not want to see them doing nothing and wasting money, do we?').

4.  Individuals and groups always appear to be 'balancing' – preserving their options with those below, securing commitment from those alongside and giving confidence to those above. At a time of difficulty or impasse, however, communication tends to be up and down the structure rather than across. In such circumstances (e.g. blocking of divisions' proposals), the division may feel it wise to heighten its activity by making direct contact with the chairman of the health authority, the regional medical officer, or some other perceived ally.

5.  'A week is a long time in politics.' Unlike the rational and organisational models, the political model plays heavily on opportunism. It is, however, a form of opportunism that must be distinguished from risk taking. Any opportunities taken need to be considered safe, but must be taken quickly. Medical committees wishing to reallocate beds may have refrained from so doing because of the implications to a long-serving and well-respected colleague but, when his untimely death is announced at the medical committee, the subject of reallocation of beds will almost certainly be raised. An orthopaedic division must watch out for opportunities which require speedy response. A DHSS handout of funds to reduce waiting lists is an obvious example, but funding which is apparently specifically earmarked can be cunningly obtained. Expenditure allocated for shared use by NHS and local government, authorities may even be a possibility (it was called joint funding!). Opportunism, whilst emanating from a position of safety, can also be artificially created by various ploys which bring about the

conditions of performance failure referred to earlier, thereby encouraging the organisation to learn more quickly. Tactics include threatening or undertaking exposure to the press, television, members of Parliament, CHCs, or by holding public meetings for waiting list cases. These tactics are not over-used because of the danger of a back-fire. Even quite rational people can react to public meetings of waiting list patients in front of television cameras and decide that orthopaedics, far from receiving additional resources, will move further down the list.

Each of the three caricatures is clearly inadequate and indeed the organisational and political models are merely deviations from the rational model. The three assumptions I have chosen to describe are really three in one and other observers might well choose different models. Whilst these three models are inadequate, they are often much closer to our assumptions about individual and organisational behaviour than we are prepared to admit. The reason for this may be that they contribute to an identikit picture which, although not completely accurate, is not far from the truth.

## Changing Attitudes

Those of us working in the Health Service can all too easily degenerate into a mood of introspective self-pity and defeat. There are two very important reasons to be more optimistic. Firstly, the NHS is not alone in facing problems of change and that ought to encourage us to some extent. Other organisations have standard operating procedures which go sadly wrong, but they still survive. The United States Air Force had an automatic response system which meant that, in a time of crisis, military aircraft be moved to the safety of civil airports. A very laudable procedure, except that during the Cuban missile crisis this meant that some aircraft were moved *nearer* to the Cuban missiles – indeed specifically into their range. Perhaps one more terrifying but consoling example – even a man with the charisma of John F. Kennedy, at a time when his position was called the most powerful in the Western world, found that his explicit instructions to remove nuclear missiles from Turkey had been ignored. Two written instructions of the President, supported by Congress, were disregarded. Perhaps the Secretary of State for Health and Social Security can take heart from this example, when he finds his words of wisdom are ignored and that he is virtually unknown to those at the work-force. Perhaps we can learn that major organisational problems are not exclusively NHS territory.

Secondly, problems are regularly discovered, confronted and solved by clinicians and administrators up and down the country all the time. The vast range of provision and performance, and the changes that regularly occur in provision and performance, are a testament to that fact. We need to recognise that changing attitudes are a prerequisite for changing behaviour.

Howells[75] outlines three characteristic patterns of change – evolutionary, expressive and explosive. The three merge into a continuum. The evolution of attitudes is extended over long periods of time involving considerable debate and argument. Attitudes about forms of punishment change – we no longer hang common thieves in England. Hospital attitudes move with society, even if with great reluctance. Separate dining rooms for different grades and groups of staff, at one time normal, are now unusual. Explosive or violent changes of attitude, at the other extreme, are illustrated by the intense pressures of brain-washing, or the stirrings of emotional oratory. The better use of hospital beds is unlikely to be influenced by such techniques, and attitude changes in this area are more likely to be achieved by controlled expression. This allows the release of any aggression followed by a more moderate attitude susceptible to reasoned modification.

One attempt to examine both the mechanics of and the attitudes towards admission procedures was published by Fairey.[49 50] This work and that of Crawford[34] suggest that there is a latent potential for improving hospital staffs' imagination, ingenuity, and energy which is waiting for release. By providing the opportunity for staff to express their views, not only do ideas come forward, but activity to resolve problems commences and attitudes begin to change. Revans[120] further suggests that, where an openness of communication exists, staff morale improves and patient stay is shortened. His striking data may require careful handling and many suggest that no cause and effect relationship is proven, but the work nevertheless does suggest that there is a potential for improvement in bed use through deliberate attention to the psychosocial factors of hospital management. In general there is a dearth of literature regarding the attitudes of staff towards the use and improved use of hospital beds. Why is this the case? Is it because the techniques or tactics are so obvious and well-known that there is no need to publish? Are the tactics so devious that it would be embarrassing to publish? Do those who have the secrets wish to keep them to themselves or are there no such secrets? Most of the attempts to change attitudes that I have observed tend to be at best indirect and at worst devious. This may be a reflection on the many clinicians with whom I have worked, but is more likely to be due to my systematically distorted observation.

Perhaps I would be alone in choosing to question a surgeon on the length of stay of his patients while negotiating with him a narrow traverse in thick cloud on a climbing expedition? Nevertheless, the many tactics used by clinicians to alter their colleagues' attitudes do become familiar after a few years of observation. The following list may provide a new meaning for the term standard deviation, but change in attitude and behaviour is not an entirely rational process!

## Removing pressure

The people, the place, the timing and the context are all important factors in changing attitudes and thereby influencing behaviour, and various steps can often be taken to improve channels of communication: an admired colleague who does not share the prejudices of the involved parties is helpful in an intermediary capacity; the initial concentration of debate on areas of common ground in order to build up trust and good relationships before moving on to main problems areas; the use of different settings and atmosphere, e.g. the bar, the changing room, a lunch table, the post-graduate or university teaching environment in preference to the committee room or the telephone conversation. All these are examples of a soft approach which seeks and maintains common ground and avoids the type of confrontation which might lead to the adoption of defensive postures. The latter can occur particularly in open formal meetings which frequently include the presentation of undiscussed and unrequested 'hard' information.

## Using pressure

Those who are in a position to improve the use of hospital beds are confronted by all sorts of pressures, many of which have little or no direct bearing on the use of beds. Some of these pressures will require changes in attitude and behaviour and such changes in one area can be used to bring along changes in another area. Changes in location, from an old to a new hospital, even from one ward to another, changes in senior staffing and shortages of staff or finances can all be used to encourage changes in the use of hospital beds. Within an overall strategy of seeking improved use of hospital beds it is possible to select opportunities to examine problems and influence attitudes as events occur. In a climate of financial difficulty, many clinicians find that their only option is to review current practice critically to see if money can be

saved for highly desirable expansion or even the desperate maintenance of their present standards and level of service. Painful incentives
are often more forceful than intellectual challenges. It may not be
morally defensible deliberately to introduce financial shortages in
order to change attitudes, but when such opportunities arise surely
they cannot be ignored.

### Creating pressure

When the so-called rational attempts at intellectual debate have failed
to produce changes in attitude, there remains the option of force, and
the forcefulness of bargaining and the subtlety of peer persuasion are
very powerful influences on attitude and thus on behaviour. Bargains
are struck in and out of committee. 'Yes, we will reduce our allocation
of beds and give them to your division, providing your division ensures
full consultant cover for emergency admissions and each consultant
always carries a 'bleep' in order that contact can be made.'

Pressure can be created by agreeing to study a situation. Such studies
can have remarkable effects on attitude and performance. Earlier (p.
42) I described how clerical staff had changed the accuracy and completeness of their performance during a period of study. McColl[94] has
described how an investigational study appeared to alter the rate of
laparotomy wound dehiscence. There is little published evidence that
studies are mounted with the deliberate intent of effecting a change in
performance but, clearly, it is a useful strategy.

CASE STUDY

A medical executive committee chairman was wrestling with the
problems of locating eight additional beds for gynaecology within a
district general hospital. Representatives of all divisions agreed that additional beds were required and the administration and management
services advice also indicated the need for additional provision. All divisions claimed they were unable to help solve the problem. The reasons
were either that all beds were fully used or that for a mixture of structu-
ral, geographical and clinical reasons there could be no mixing of
specialties on wards which had vacant beds. Many of the consultants felt
that the surgical division had not been as cooperative as it might have
been. Throughout the debate its representatives adamantly denied any
spare capacity. Eventually the physicians agreed in a private discussion
with the chairman of the MEC and the gynaecologists that six beds
could be provided on a female medical ward for a trial period throughout the summer months. All parties to the agreement expressed concern
about the lack of cooperation from the surgeons and decided that they
would not make the new agreement public until a further debate could
be arranged with the surgeons to examine the surgical work-load and

bed use. The MEC then pressed the surgical division to agree to a three-month prospective survey of surgical activity to ascertain whether surgical wards had the capacity to share facilities with gynaecology. After the three-month study, comparison of data was made with that from similar periods. Discharges and deaths increased by over 15% and empty beds declined from 25% to 15%. The surgeons were delighted to demonstrate that they had no spare capacity, but their colleagues were delighted to see an increase in activity even if only short-lived.

Change in performance can only be achieved when attitudes also change. Attitudes are resistant to change;[75] our task is to ensure that changes are made quickly and for the better. In order to do this we need a collection of analytical and behavioural skills, but above all we need to be able to judge which skill is appropriate to a given situation.

## Prognosis and Advice

Chapter 2 outlined some of the principal dysfunctions, or 'diseases' found when examining the amount, use, and spare capacity of hospital beds. It is likely that, in the next decade, the overall amount of bed stock will decrease and unless efforts are made to reallocate within the existing stock, reduce the steadily increasing amount of spare capacity, and reconsider the way in which occupied beds are used, then the outlook is likely to be one of increasing waiting lists and waiting time for cold surgery with an increasing likelihood of patients dying before admission. Confronting the dysfunctions with which we are faced, the resistance to change which we encounter will require a thorough analysis of the problems faced, the solutions suggested, and – equally important – the motivations present. To improve the use of our hospital beds we must be more scientific in our approach to the problems faced and yet at the same time recognise the reality of the uncharted waters of organisational behaviour. Those seeking such improvements need to develop a broad strategy which might be outlined as follows:

1. Undertake a rational analysis of the problems you are faced with in order to satisfy yourself of the merits and demerits of any action you propose.
2. Make the problem explicit to others, even if you think it is already obvious.
3. Recognise that more resources in one area means less for another. This may force you to demonstrate not only the merits of one particular case, but its merits *vis-à-vis* other cases.

4. Be prepared to participate in demonstrating how resources can be saved outside your own area.

5. Familiarise yourself with the mechanics of your organisation – you do not want to fail on a technicality.

6. Get to know who you are dealing with and ensure that they know you personally and are aware of the issues you are facing.

7. Look for allies who are prepared to share scarce resources with you.

# *Appendix*

# *The Barber-Johnson Diagram*

## Introduction

In 1973, Barber and Johnson[11] described a method of presenting information about patient length of stay, turnover interval, discharges and deaths per available bed and percentage bed occupancy, on one diagram. At first sight the diagram appears complex, but it has the advantage of showing how the four variables are related. The technique is not widely used and this appendix is included in order to publicise the technique and discuss its values and limitations. This description includes some small modifications in presentation but the basic method remains unchanged.

## The Basic Figures and Calculated Variables

Three basic figures about the use of hospital beds are the number of *available beds*, the number of *beds occupied*, and the number of *discharges and deaths*. These three figures are to be found on the annual statistical forms SH3 and other quarterly returns completed for each hospital in England and Wales. It is from these three basic figures that a number of variables can be calculated. Barber and Johnson selected four variables: length of stay; turnover interval; discharges and deaths per available bed; and percentage bed occupancy, for presentation on their diagram. I have chosen to replace bed occupancy by bed emptiness. The four variables can be calculated for a year from the basic figures as follows:

If  A = Available beds (expressed as an average for the year)
    O = Occupied beds (average for year)
    D = Discharges and deaths (number for year)

then,

*Average length of stay* (LOS; expressed in days) becomes:

$$LOS = \frac{O \times 365}{D}$$

This is a shorthand method of estimating the length of stay which effectively sums all the occupied bed days in a period and divides that figure by the number of discharges and deaths in the same period. This is not necessarily the same average as that of the actual stay of all patients discharged during the period, but in acute specialties with a reasonable number of patients it is usually a sufficiently accurate figure. The figure appears on form SH3 and thus saves the need for calculation.

*Average turnover interval* (TOI; expressed in days)

$$TOI = \frac{(A - O) \times 365}{D}$$

This is the average time that beds are left empty between each discharge and admission. It might be better understood as the average length of emptiness. This figure does not appear on the form SH3.

*Average number of discharges and deaths per available bed* (DDPB; expressed as a number per year):

$$DDPB = \frac{D}{A}$$

This becomes a measure of throughput or activity. The simplicity of the calculation should not obscure the fact that the figure of available beds (A) is composed of both length of stay and turnover interval. Throughput must not be seen merely as a function of length of stay – it also includes the turnover interval. The average number of discharges and deaths per available bed appears on form SH3.

*Average bed emptiness* (expressed as a percentage):

$$\% \text{ Empt.} = \frac{(A - O) \times 100}{A}$$

This is a crude description of unused capacity. NB: Barber and Johnson used percentage occupancy rather than percentage emptiness. (Neither average bed emptiness nor occupancy appear on form SH3.)

## A Description of the Diagram

In Fig. A, the horizontal and vertical lines are turnover interval and length of stay respectively. Figure B adds the percentage emptiness lines that radiate from the origin. In Fig. C, points on each axis are joined and the resultant diagonal lines show the number of discharges and deaths per available bed (sometimes abbreviated to 'throughput'). The closer such lines are to the origin, the higher the throughput.

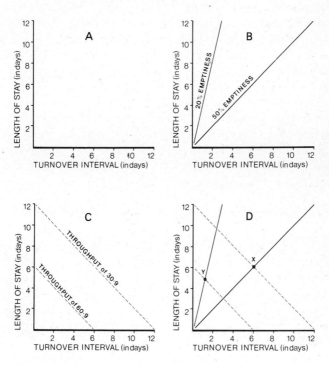

Constructing a
BARBER-JOHNSON diagram

Figs A–D

Putting the three diagrams together produces Fig. D. One point on the diagram now gives four figures. Point X has a 6·0-day length of stay, a 6·0-day turnover interval, 50% bed emptiness, and a throughput of 30·4 patients per available bed. It can be seen that to move from point X towards point Y will involve changes in all four variables. LOS and TOI will be shorter, percentage emptiness will decrease, and throughput will increase. We cannot change one single variable without altering at least two other variables.

## Constructing the Diagram

The first four figures were constructed with a ratio of one to one between the scales adopted for length of stay and turnover interval. Whilst this ratio can be used for plotting the Barber–Johnson diagram, the plotting of acute specialty activity usually results in the clustering of figures on one side of the graph and, to provide a more balanced diagram, a ratio of two days' length of stay to one day of turnover interval is recommended. A graph with 20 days' length of stay on the vertical axis and 10 days' turnover interval on the horizontal axis covers most acute specialty activity. The new shape of the diagram appears in Fig. E. The presentation of the diagram can be aided by ensuring that the percentage emptiness and throughput lines are marked in a separate manner from the two axes.

Unless detailed work is intended, the only variables which require numbers to be precisely plotted are length of stay (already on SH3 forms) and turnover interval. The other two variables can be read approximately from the diagram, provided a sufficient number of lines have been plotted. The marking of the percentage emptiness and throughput lines can be done as follows:

| For a percentage emptiness of: | plot a point that joins a length of stay of: | with a turnover interval of: | and draw a line through that point to the origin. |
|---|---|---|---|
| 90% | 1·0 | 9 | |
| 80% | 2·0 | 8 | |
| 70% | 3·0 | 7 | |
| 60% | 4·0 | 6 | |
| 50% | 5·0 | 5 | |
| 45% | 5·5 | 4·5 | |
| 40% | 6·0 | 4 | |
| 30% | 7·0 | 3 | |
| 25% | 7·5 | 2·5 | |
| 20% | 8·0 | 2 | |
| 15% | 8·5 | 1·5 | |
| 10% | 9·0 | 1 | |
| 5% | 9·5 | 0·5 | |

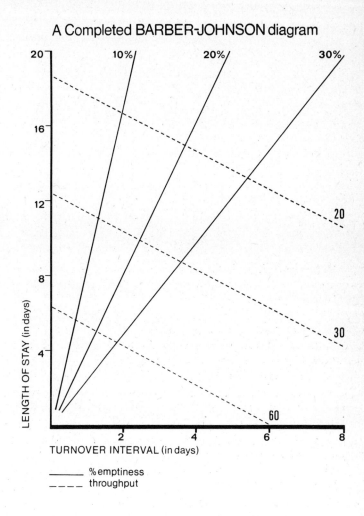

Fig. E

To plot the throughput lines on the graph, the following method is suggested;

| For a throughput of: | join the following points on the length of stay axis with the same points on the turnover interval axis: |
|---|---|
| 80 | 4·56 |
| 60 | 6·08 |
| 50 | 7·30 |
| 40 | 9·13 |
| 35 | 10·43 |
| 30 | 12·17 |
| 25 | 14·60 |
| 20 | 18·26 |
| 15 | 24·33 |
| 10 | 36·50 |

## Using the Diagram

The diagram can be used for checking the statistical calculations which appear on SH3 and similar forms but its principal value lies in its use as an explanatory and comparative tool.

### Checking calculations
The known relationship between the four variables enables quick cross-checking of some of the information on SH3 forms and similar statistical information. If three or four of the figures presented do not produce one point on the diagram then an error exists in at least one of the figures.

A second check is that of figures against feelings. A discussion of the variables on the diagram with a clinician from the hospital or specialty concerned can help even a relatively unskilled interpreter of statistics to know whether the information contains glaring anomalies (e.g. false bed availability).

A third way of looking for errors is to plot information for each year of a five-year period. In most specialties the five points on the graph will appear in the same area of the diagram. Any point which is some distance away from the others may be explained by a change of clinical policy or bed availability but may also indicate an error in information collection or calculation. (This method of error detection is illustrated below under the heading of comparison over time.)

**Explaining relationships between the variables**

The diagram helps to describe the relationship between the four variables displayed. As an example, one can consider the desire which is often expressed that acute hospitals or units should make better use of the beds available despite having a short length of stay. By examining Fig. E, it can be seen that a specialty which has a length of stay of four days cannot be expected to achieve a 10% bed emptiness level unless a very low (almost impracticable) turnover interval is achieved. On the other hand, if a turnover interval of two days is considered reasonable, then a bed emptiness level of over 30% must be expected. The plotting of four variables on the one diagram can help one understand the difficulties encountered, especially by short-stay specialties, in attaining a low emptiness of the beds provided.

The explanatory properties of the diagram are helpful in predicting the consequences of changes of policy (e.g. a deliberate policy to shorten stay or increase throughput) or of changing provision (e.g. assessing the effect of providing additional or fewer beds). For those who wish to embark on shortening stay without increasing emptiness, the diagram will explain that this can only be achieved by improving throughput and also demonstrates how much throughput will be required for given reductions in stay.

**Comparison of activity patterns**

1. *Comparison over time*

Figure F shows the performance of a general medical unit over a five-year period. The first three years have some consistency but years 1976 and 1977 show comparatively lower lengths of stay and higher throughput emptiness and turnover intervals. In this case the explanation is that the three physicians appointed early in 1976 have a different policy from that of their predecessors.

Also appearing in Fig. F is the performance of a thoracic surgical unit over the same five years. In 1975 the turnover interval moved to over eight days compared with the figure of about 4·5 days for other years. This surprising movement (not due to industrial action) appeared to warrant further investigation and it was discovered that the bed availability figure for 1975 had been incorrectly calculated. This illustrates the error-checking capability referred to earlier.

In Chapter 4, Fig. 8 attempted to illustrate the quarterly activity of an ophthalmological unit over a period of three years. Successive quarters were joined up by lines with arrows to show the direction of

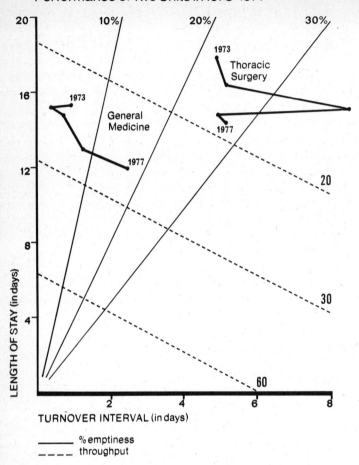

Fig. F

change. The unit was working under very little pressure until the closure of a nearby hospital forced more work onto the unit. Following the reopening of the nearby hospital, the specialty began to return to its original work-load, but a change in consultant appointment resulted in a second change of direction.

2. *Comparison between units* (specialties, hospitals or districts)
Figure G plots the performance of four paediatric and four general surgical units. The overall figure for England and Wales in each spe-

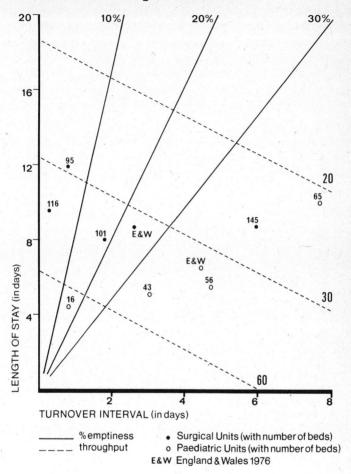

A Comparison of Four Paediatric and
Four General Surgical Units 1976

Fig. G

cialty is also shown. As would be expected, length of stay in paediatrics is shorter than in general surgery, but ranges of approximately 4 – 9 days in paediatrics and 8 – 12 days in general surgery can be seen. The wide range of turnover intervals (0·2 – 7·7 days) is interesting. In this case this difference cannot be explained by errors in the figures. Points to the extreme left-hand side of the diagram are likely to indicate that allocations are inadequate for current policies (without commenting on whether those policies are correct). Points on the right-hand side of the diagram would indicate that bed allocation is higher than necessary or, alternatively, higher than use of other facilities (e.g. staffing, diagnostic facilities, theatres, etc.) will permit. A more comprehensive comparison is shown in Fig. H, which illustrates the performance of 202 health districts in England in 1977 for traumatic and orthopaedic surgery. The interpretation of this diagram is susceptible to many reservations, nevertheless, large variations across the country are seen to exist.

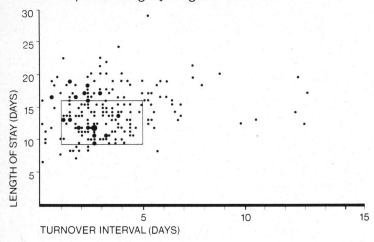

Scattergram
Length of Stay against Turnover Interval: by District
Orthopædic Surgery: England 1977

Fig. H

### 3. *Comparisons against agreed standards*

It is possible to place on the diagram a 'zone' in which activity of a unit or units could reasonably be expected to fall. This method is illustrated in Fig. H, but could also be used for studying one unit's performance over time. In Fig. H the zone of expected performance was chosen by a group of senior orthopaedic surgeons in advance of the data being made available to them. All of the surgeons concerned found that their own unit was within the zone chosen, but they were surprised to see the number of units not in the expected ranges covered by the zone. The agreement of zones by staff before seeing where their unit appears on the diagram can produce interesting reactions. It is also worth noting that prospective rather than retrospective agreements are generally found to produce more debate, commitment and action.

All three of the comparative methods described above can be used to initiate or enlighten debate on bed use within and between specialties. Whilst comparisons can be odious, they can also be instructive, albeit painfully so. The diagram cannot successfully be placed before a complete medical committee unless all members are conversant with the variables and the method, but its use by individual clinicians and small groups of clinicians has frequently stimulated debate – sometimes heated, sometimes enlightened – and such debate can lead to action.

## Points to Watch

1. The diagram will be valueless if the basic information is incorrect. The figure of bed availability is particularly apt to nullify the value of the diagram if it is incorrect. The recording of this figure in hospitals can be poor. Short-term closures because of infection, ward decoration, etc. are often missed and paper figures of additional beds long since taken away often continue unnoticed. Five-day wards can even be credited with a seven-day availability according to SH3 rules. Moreover, it is doubtful whether the midnight census is representative of bed-occupancy in very short-stay, high-turnover wards, and it should also be noted that the separation of day-cases from other discharges is not always undertaken accurately.

2. All four variables are expressed as an average (arithmetic mean) which can be a poor descriptive tool. Before making policy decisions from the information presented on the diagram, the distribution of the average of each variable should be understood.

3. The size of units is not discernible from the diagram unless marked (e.g. in Fig. G). In order to compare two different units or one unit over time one should refer to bed availability figures. Comparisons need to distinguish between units of 3 bed and those of 103, as both could appear on the same part of the diagram.

4. Small numbers (available beds or number of discharges and deaths) may be the cause of considerable variations when calculating the four variables. Violent fluctuations on the diagram can occur in small specialties or when larger specialties are plotted for short periods of, say, one month.

5. One small point to be noted is that the original paper was con-

ceived when the SH3 ruling on bed availability was such that borrowed beds were not reduced from the specialty from which the beds were being borrowed and this meant that the borrowing specialty could achieve bed occupancies in excess of 100% and negative turnover intervals. This accounted for the original form of diagram. This state of affairs no longer exists (according to SH3 rules!). The matter was clarified in later correspondence.[80 107 108]

6.  The diagram can be helpful in identifying areas for further investigation. It does not make value judgements.

## Acknowledgements

My thanks go to Barry Barber, Brian Cook and Michael Davidge for their help in my studies of this technique.

# References

1. Abel-Smith B. (Chairman) (1973). *Accounting for Health*. Report of a working party on the application of economic principles to health service management. King Edward's Hospital Fund for London.
2. Ackoff R. L., Emery F. E. (1972). *On Purposeful Systems*. London: Tavistock Publications.
3. Allison G. T. (1971). *Essence of Decision*. Boston: Little Brown.
4. Anscombe A. R., Hancock B. D., Humphreys W. V. (1974). A clinical trial of the treatment of haemorrhoids by operation and the Lord procedure. *Lancet; 2:* 250–253.
5. Asher R. A. J. (1947). The dangers of going to bed. *Br.Med.J; 2:* 967–968.
6. Ashford J. R. (1977). Planning local health services. In *Framework and Design for Planning* (McLachlan G., ed.). Oxford University Press for Provincial Hospitals Trust.
7. Ashley J. S. A. (1972). Present state of statistics from hospital in-patient data and their uses. *Br.J.Prev.Soc.Med.; 26:* 135–147.
8. Ashley J. S. A., Klein R. E. (1971). The challenge of another million by 1991. *Mod.Geriat.; 1:* 310.
9. Avery Jones F. (1964). Length of stay in hospital. *Lancet; 1:* 321–322.
10. Baderman H., Corless C., Fairey M. J., Modell M., Ramsden Y. (1973). *Admission of Patients to Hospital*. King Edward's Hospital Fund for London.
11. Barber B., Johnson D. (1973). The presentation of acute hospital in-patient statistics. *Hospital and Health Services Review; 69:* 11–14.
12. Barker D. J. P., Rose G. (1976). *Epidemiology in Medical Practice*. Edinburgh: Churchill Livingstone.
13. Bates T., Menzies K., Behr A., Rendall M. (1976). The place of early social assessment in the management of surgical patients. *Postgrad.Med.J.; 52:* 61–65.
14. Bell J. R., Shearer D. S. (1972). Economic use of hospital beds. *Nursing Times, 68:* 1264–1265.
15. Benjamin B. (1965). Hospital Activity Analysis. An information feed-back for the consultant. *The Hospital 61:* 221–228.
16. Bennett A. E. (1966). Case selection in a London teaching hospital. *Medical Care; 4:* 138–141.

17. Beresford S. A. A., Chant A. D. P., Piachaud D.,Weddell J. M., Jones H. O. (1978). Varicose veins: a comparison of surgery and injection compression sclerotherapy; five year follow-up. *Lancet; 1:* 921–924.

18. Bithell J. F. (1969). A survey of in-patients of a London teaching hospital: general results. *Br.J.Prev.Soc.Med.; 23:* 101–105.

19. Bithell J. F., Devlin H. B. (1968). Prediction of discharge of hospital inpatients. *Health Services Research; 3:* 174–184.

20. Boardman K. P., Griffiths J. C. (1977). Elective out-patient surgery in orthopaedics. *Health Trends; 9:* 9–11.

21. British Medical Journal (1974). Five day wards in 1974 (leading article). *Br.Med.J; 2:* 71–72.

22. Burgess C., Chant A. D. B., Beschi J. (1978). Elective surgery and a programmed investigation unit in a five day ward. *Hospital and Health Services Review; 75:* 427–428.

23. Burn J. M. B. (1976). Preoperative assessment clinics. *Proc.Roy.Soc.Med.; 69:* 734–736.

24. Calnan J. (1977). Staying out of hospital. *World Medicine; 13:* 38–39.

25. Calnan J., Barabas A. (1972). *Speaking at Medical Meetings – a Practical Guide.* London: William Heinemann Medical Books.

26. Calnan J., Barabas A. (1973). *Writing Medical Papers – a Practical Guide.* London: William Heinemann Medical Books.

27. Carstairs V., Heasman M. A. (1974). The hospital: towards a rational use. *Br.Med.Bull.; 30:* 228–233.

28. Chant A. D. P., Napier M. (1973). Factors influencing prediction of surgical in-patient stay. *Hospital and Health Services Review; 69:* 52–54.

29. Chant A. D. P., McGinn F. P., Triger D. R., Wales J. M. (1975). Hospital bed: a method for evaluating their use. Hospital and Health Services Review; 71: 263–265.

30. Chubb P. L., Hodgkinson A. (1974). A bed information system for district general hospitals. *Hospital and Health Services Review; 70:* 127–129.

31. Clayton S. G., Feroze R. M., Brudenall J. M., Burt J., Sanderson B. W., Beard R. W. (1971). Short-stay gynaecology ward. *Lancet; 2:* 1197–1198.

32. Cochrane A. L. (1972). *Effectiveness and Efficiency.* Nuffield Provincial Hospitals Trust.

33. Craig G. A. (1970). Use of day beds in gynaecology. *Br.Med.J.; 2:* 786–787.

34. Crawford L. E. (1975). Hospital 'de-administration' experiences in six teaching hospitals. *Med.J.Aust.; 1:* 348–353.

35. Crosby D. L., Griffiths G. H., Jenkins J. R. E., Real R., Roberts

B. C., Forrest A. P. M. (1972). General surgical pre-admission clinic. *Br.Med.J.; 3:* 157–159.

36. Davidge M. G., Yates J. M., Wainwright L. (1981). Midnight magic? *Hospital and Health Services Review; 77:* 131–134.

37. Davies T. F. (1975). Programmed investigation bed. *Br.Med.J.; 4:* 149–150.

38. Department of Health and Social Security (1969). *Hospital Activity Analysis.* HM(69)79.

39. Department of Health and Social Security (1974). *Abstracts of Efficiency Studies in the Hospital Service.* E.N.T. Department: Increasing bed occupancy. No. 167. London: HMSO.

40. Department of Health and Social Services (1976). *Abstracts of Efficiency Studies in the National Health Service.* In-patient Arrangements: Programmed Investigation Bed. No. 174. London: HMSO.

41. Department of Health and Social Security (1976). *Abstracts of Efficiency Studies in the National Health Service.* In-patient Arrangements: Programmed Investigation and Treatment Unit. No. 175. London: HMSO.

42. Department of Health and Social Security (1977). *Notes on Hospital Form SH3 for 1977.* London: HMSO.

43. Department of Health and Social Security (1977). *Health and Personal Social Service Statistics for England.* London: HMSO.

44. Department of Health and Social Services, Office of Population Censuses and Surveys (1974). *Report on Hospital In-patient Enquiry for the Year 1972.* London: HMSO.

45. Devlin H. B. (1977). Planned early discharge. *Update; 15:* 125–133.

46. Donaldson S. N., Wheeler M. R., Barr A. (1977). Demand for patient care. *Br.Med.J.; 2:* 799–802.

47. Doran F. S. A., White M., Drury M. (1972). The scope and safety of short-stay surgery in the treatent of groin herniae and varicose veins. *Br.J.Surg.; 59:* 333–339.

48. Duthie R. B., Mullins J. L., Pace A. J. (1973). The formation of an admission unit in a specialist hospital. *Health Trends; 5:* 4–7.

49. Fairey M. J., Webster B., Barbar B. (1970). Admission procedures at a London teaching hospital – 1. *Br.J.Hosp.Med.; 2:* 804–808.

50 Fairey M. J. (1970). Admission procedures at a London teaching hospital – 2. *Ibid; 2:* 810–820.

51. Farquaharson E. L. (1955). Early ambulation with special reference to herniorrhaphy as an out-patient procedure. *Lancet; 2:* 517–519.

52. Fernow L. C., McColl I., Mackie C. (1978). Firm, patient and

process variables associated with length of stay in four diseases. *Br.Med.J.; 1:* 556–559.

53. Ferrer H. P. (1972). *The Health Services – Administration, Research and Management.* London: Butterworth.

54. Forsyth G., Logan R. F. L. (1962). Studies in medical care: an assessment of some methods. In *Towards a Measure of Medical Care.* Oxford University Press for Nuffield Provincial Hospitals Trust.

55. Friend J. H. (1978). A reorganised medical division. *Br.Med.J.; 2:* 1676–1678.

56. Gainsborough H. (1969). The myth of the acute hospital. *British Hospital Journal and Social Service Review; 79:* 447–449.

57. Gandy R. J. (1978). An evaluation of the effect of a programmed investigation unit. *Health Trends; 10:* 64–65.

58. Gardiner R. H., Moreny M. H. (1970). The reduction of the surgical waiting list. *Health Trends; 2:* 49–51.

59. Gelson A. D. N., Carson P. H. M., Tucker H. H., Phillips R., Clarke M., Oakley G. D. G. (1976). Course of patients discharged early after myocardial infarction. *Br.Med.J.; 1:* 1555–1558.

60. Gilkes M. J., Handa V. K. (1974). The duration of pre- and post-operative in-patient stay in ophthalmology. *Health Trends; 6:* 76–78.

61. Grant A. P. (1975). The problems of acute medical units in an emergency bed service. *Hospital and Health Services Review; 71:* 299–303.

62. Griffiths D. A. T. (1978). Information rooms for operational management in general hospitals. *Hospital and Health Services Review; 74:* 124–127.

63. Griffiths D. A. T. (1978). Information rooms for operational management in general hospitals – 2. *Ibid; 74:* 157–160.

64. Griffith J. R., Hancock W. M., Munson F. C. (1973). Practical ways to contain hospital costs. *Harvard Business Review; 51:* 131–139.

65. Hadaway E. G., Ingram R. M., Traynar M. J. (1977). Day case surgery for strabismus in children. *Trans.Ophthal.Soc.U.K.; 97:* 23–25.

66. Harpur J. E., Conner W. T., Hamilton M., Kellett R. J., Galbraith H. (1971). Controlled trial of early mobilisation and discharge from hospital in uncomplicated myocardial infarction. *Lancet; 2:* 1331–1334.

67. Hawkins C. F. (1964). Speaking at meetings. *Lancet; 1:* 261–263.

68. Heald R. J. (1980). Towards fewer colostomies. *Br.J.Surg.; 67:* 198–200.

69. Heasman M. A. (1964). How long in hospital? *Lancet;* 2: 539–541.
70. Heasman M. A., Carstairs V. (1971). In-patient management; variations in some aspects of practice in Scotland. *Br.Med.J.;* 1: 495–498.
71. *Herald of Wales* (1977). 28 May.
72. Hicks D. (1976). *The Management of 120-Bed Clinical Nursing Units, an Account of Research Carried Out in the Five Years 1970–1974.* Parts 1 and 2: Wessex Regional Health Authority.
73. Hill J. D., Hampton J. R., Mitchell J. R. A. (1978). A randomised trial of home-versus-hospital management for patients with suspected myocardial infarction. *Lancet;* 1: 837–841.
74. Hindle A. (1972). A practical approach to surgical scheduling. In *The Health Services – Administration, Research and Management* (Ferrer H. P., ed.). London: Butterworth.
75. Howells G. W. (1972). *Executive Aspects of Man Management.* London: Pitman.
76. Hughes A. O., Miller D. S. (1975). The determinants of demand for pre-convalescent beds. *Hospital and Health Services Review;* 71: 350–353.
77. Hunter B. (1972). *The Administration of Hospital Wards.* Manchester University Press.
78. Hutter A. M., Sidel V. W., Shine K. I., DeSanta R. W. (1973). Early hospital discharge after myocardial infarction. *New Eng.J.Med.;* 228: 1141–1144.
79. Ingram R. M., Traynar P. M. (1976). Five-and-a-half-day ophthalmic ward. *Br.Med.J.;* 1: 445–446.
80. Johnson D., Barber B. (1973). Bed utilisation (letter). *Hospital and Health Services Review;* 69: 132.
81. Keith S. (1973). The hospital in-patient enquiry 1970. *Health Trends;* 5: 13–14.
82. King D. J., Leach J. D. (1975). Assessing the capacity of a district health service to meet a local need. In *Measuring for Management* (McLachlan G., ed.). Oxford University Press for Nuffield Provincial Hospitals Trust.
83. King D. J., Court M. T. W., Leach J. D., Tarr D. (1977). An information service for planning and managing a national health service district. In *Framework and Design for Planning* (McLachlan G., ed.). Oxford University Press for Nuffield Provincial Hospitals Trust.
84. Kozak L. J., Andersen R., Anderson O. W. (1978). *Hospital Statistics in England and Wales.* University of Chicago, Centre for Health Administration Studies.
85. Lawson R. (1974). Medical Admission Policies. In *Information for Action* (Goldsmith O., Mason A., eds.). Joint Working Party

on Organisation of Medical Work in Hospitals. London: Department of Health and Social Security.

86. Lennox B., Clarke J. A., Ewen S. W. B. (1978). Incidence of salivary gland tumours in Scotland: accuracy of national records. *Br.Med.J.; 1:* 687–689.

87. Lockwood E. (1971). Accuracy of Scottish hospital morbidity data. *Br.J.Prev.Soc.Med.; 25:* 76–83.

88. Logan R. F. L., Ashley J. S. A., Klein R. E., Robson D. M. (1972). *Dynamics of Medical Care.* Memoir no.14, London School of Hygiene and Tropical Medicine.

89. Longson D., Young B. (1973). The Manchester Royal Infirmary programmed investigation unit. *Br.Med.J.; 4:* 528–531.

90. Loudon I. S. L. (1970). *The Demand for Hospital Care.* United Oxford Hospitals, The Radcliffe Infirmary, Oxford.

91. Luck G. M., Luckman J., Smith B. W., Stringer J. (1971). *Patients, Hospitals, and Operational Research.* Tavistock Publications.

92. Luckman J., Murray F. (1972). The health programme of the Institute for Operational Research, – 3 Management policies for a gynaecology department. *Health Trends; 2:* 33–38.

93. McArdle C., Wylie J. C., Alexander W. D. (1975). Geriatric patients in an acute medical ward. *Br.Med.J.; 4:* 568–569.

94. McColl I. (1976). Observations on the quality of surgical care. In *A Question of Quality* (McLachlan G., ed.). Oxford University Press for Nuffield Provincial Hospitals Trust.

95. McKeown T. (1976). *The Role of Medicine, Dream, Mirage or Nemesis?* Nuffield Provincial Hospitals Trust.

96. McNay R. A. (1969). Hospital Activity Analysis: experience in the area of the Newcastle Regional Hospital Board. *The Hospital. 65:* 308–312.

97. McNeilly R. H., Moore F. (1975). The accuracy of some Hospital Activity Analysis data. *Hospital and Health Services Review; 71:* 93–95.

98. Marshall R. D., Spencer R. I. (1974). A more efficient use of hospital beds? *Br.Med.J.; 3:* 27–30.

99. Martindale B. V., Garfield J. (1978). Subarachnoid haemorrhage above the age of 59: are intracranial investigations justified? *Br.Med.J.; 1:* 465–466.

100. Martini C. J. M., Hughes A. O., Patton V. A. (1976). A study of the validity of the Hospital Activity Analysis information. *Brit.J.Prev.Soc.Med.; 30:* 180–186.

101. Mather H. G., Pearson N. G., Read K. L. Q., Shaw D. B., Steed G. R., Thorne M. G., Jones S., Guerrier C. J., Eraut C. D., McHugh P. M., Chowdhury N. R., Jafary M. H., Wallace T. J.

(1971). Acute myocardial infarction: home and hospital treatment. *Br.Med.J.; 3:* 334–338.

102. Mather H. G., Morgan D. C., Pearson N. G., Read K. L. Q., Shaw D. B., Steed C. R., Thorne M. G., Lawrence C. J., Riley I. S., (1976). Myocardial infarction: a comparison between home and hospital care for patients. *Br.Med.J.; 2:* 925–929.
103. Mawson S. R., Stroud C. E. (1972). The indications for tonsillectomy and adenoidectomy. *Health Trends; 4:* 31–32.
104. Meredith J. S., Anderson M. A., Price A. C., Leithead J. (1968). *'Hostels' in Hospitals?* Oxford University Press for Nuffield Provincial Hospitals Trust.
105. Ministry of Health (1957). *Hospital In-patient Enquiry.* HM(57)56.
106. Ministry of Health (1967). *1st Report of the Joint Working Party on the Organisation of Medical Work in Hospitals.* London: HMSO.
107. Morris D. (1973). Bed utilisation statistics (letter). *Hospital and Health Services Review; 69:* 104.
108. Morris D. (1973). Bed utilisation statistics (letter). *Ibid; 69:* 306.
109. Morris D., Handyside A. J. (1971). Effects of methods of admitting emergencies on use of hospital beds. *Br.J.Prev.Soc.Med.; 25:* 1–11.
110. Morris D., Buckler M., Goss F., Harvie J., Williams R., Willox I. (1974). *Cogstats.* King Edward's Fund for London.
111. Murphy F. W. (1977). Blocked beds. *Br.Med.J.; 2:* 1395–1396.
112. Murray F. A., Topley L. (1974). H.A.A. and SH3 information systems in function. *Health and Social Service Journal; 84:* 2652–2653.
113. Newell D. J. (1954). Provision of emergency beds in hospitals. *Br.J.Prev.Soc.Med.; 8:* 77–80.
114. Nicoll J. H. (1909). The surgery of infancy. *Br.Med.J.; 2:* 753–754.
115. Oxford Regional Hospital Board (1966). *More use from available beds.* Operational Research Unit.
116. Parkin D. M., Clarke J. A., Heasman M. A. (1976). Scottish consultant review of in-patient statistics (SCRIPS). *Health Bulletin; 34:* 273–278.
117. Parkin D. M., Clarke J. A., Heasman M. A. (1976). Routine statistical data for the clinician. Review and prospect. *Health Bulletin; 34:* 279–284.
118. Pike M. C., Proctor D. M., Wyllie J. M. (1963). Analysis of admission to a casualty ward. *Br.J.Prev.Soc.Med; 17:* 172–176.
119. Ramsey T. A. (1965). New district hospitals. Problems associ-

ated with assessing the need and the facilities required. *The Hospital* (London); *61:* 345–348.

120. Revans R. W. (1976). *Action Learning in Hospitals.* Maidenhead: McGraw-Hill.
121. Rhodes P. (1976). *Value of Medicine.* London: Allen and Unwin.
122. Rohde P. D. (1973). Hospital Activity Analysis statistics. *Br.Med.J.; 3:* 351–352.
123. Royal College of Physicians (1975). The care of the patient with coronary heart disease. Report of a Joint Working Party of the Royal College of Physicians of London and the British Cardiac Society. *J.Roy.Coll.Physns.; 10:* 5–46.
124. Royal Commission on the NHS (1978). *Management of Financial Resources in the NHS.* Research Paper no.2. London: HMSO.
125. Rowe R. G., Brewer W. (1972). *Hospital Activity Analysis.* London: Butterworth.
126. Rubin S. G., Davies G. H. (1975). Bed blocking by elderly patients in general hospital wards. *Age and Ageing; 4:* 142–147.
127. Ruckley C. V. (1978). Day care and short stay surgery for hernia. *Br.J.Surg.; 65:* 1–4.
128. Russell I. T., Devlin H. B., Fell M., Glass N. J., Newell D. J. (1977). Day case surgery for hernias and haemorrhoids. A clinical, social and economic evaluation. *Lancet; 1:* 844–846.
129. Sachdev Y., Gomez-Pan A., Fletcher P. M., Hall R. (1976). Programmed investigation unit. *Br.Med.J.; 2:* 91–93.
130. Schnurr L. P., Geddes A. M., Ball A. P., Gray J., McGhie D. (1977). Bacterial endocartitis in England in the 1970's. A review of 70 patients. *Quarterly J.Med.; XLVI:* 499–512.
131. Simpson J. E. P. (1977). Length of stay. *Lancet; 2:* 531–533.
132. Simpson J. E. P., Cox A. G., Meade T. W., Brennan P. J. (1977). "Right" stay in hospital after surgery: randomised controlled trial. *Br.Med.J.; 2:* 1514–1516.
133. Southam J. A., Talbot R. W. (1980). Planned surgical admissions in a district hospital. *Br.Med.J.; 1:* 808–809.
134. Spencer R. I. (1974). Determining waiting list admissions. *Hospital and Health Services Review; 70:* 308–311.
135. Strang I. W., Boddy F. A., Jennett, B. (1977). Patients in acute surgical wards: a survey in Glasgow. *Br.Med.J.; 1:* 545–548.
136. Sutton A. (1973). *Functions of an Orthopaedic Unit Information Room.* No. 728. London: Institute for Operational Research.
137. Todd J. W. (1977). The use of hospitals, 2. The short-term inpatient. *Hospital Update; 3:* 411–416.
138. Towers M. K. (1974). Five day wards in 1974 (letter). *Br.Med.J.; 2:* 439.

139. Wagman H., Bamford D. S. (1973). Minor gynaecological out-patient operations. *Br.Med.J.; 1:* 450–451.
140. Weir M. (1978). Balancing resources for more effective use: an assessment of bed and theatre allocation. In *Management Services and the Clinician*. Harrogate Seminar Reports 2. DHSS.
141. West R. J. (1978). Determination of specialty catchment areas using H.A.A.. *Hospital and Health Services Review; 74:* 10–12.
142. West R. R., Carey M. J. (1978). Variations in the rates of hospital admission for appendicitis in Wales. *Br.Med.J.; 1:* 1662–1664.
143. Wilkes J. S., Lockhart M. P. (1974). Reviewing the bed usage in a children's hospital – a case study in operational research. *Health Bulletin; XXXIII:* 70–73.
144. Williams B. (1968). The use and misuse of bed-occupancy and waiting-list figures. *Lancet; 1:* 1029–1030.
145. Willis A. T., Ferguson I. R., Jones P. H., Phillips K. D., Tearle P. V., Berry R. B., Fiddian R. V., Graham D. F., Harland D. H. C., Innes D. B., Mee W. M., Rothwell-Jackson R. L., Sutch I., Kilbey C., Edwards D. (1976). Metronidazole in the prevention and treatment of bacteroides infections after appendicectomy. *Br.Med.J.; 1:* 318–321.
146. Wood S. K., Sutton A., Allen E. (1974). Admission policies for a 120 bedded ward unit. In *Information for Action* (Goldsmith O., Mason A., eds.). Joint Working Party on Organisation of Medical Work in Hospitals: London: Department of Health and Social Security.
147. Woodward R. H., Goldsmith P. L. (1964). *Cumulative sum techniques*. Monograph no. 3: Oliver and Boyd for I.C.I. Ltd.
148. Wynne J., Hull D. (1977). Why are children admitted to hospital? *Br.Med.J.; 4:* 1140–1142.
149. Yates J. M. (1974). An experiment in monitoring work-load. In *Information for Action* (Goldsmith O., Mason A., eds.). Joint Working Party on the Organisation of Medical Work in Hospitals. London: Department of Health and Social Security.
150. Yates J. M. (1980). *Waiting for Hospital Treatment*. Harrogate Seminar Paper July 1978: London: Department of Health and Social Security.
151. Yates J. M., Vickerstaff L. (1982). Monitoring mental handicap hospitals. *APEX Journal of British Institute of Mental Handicap*. (in press).
152. Zinovieff A., Newell D. J., Hunt L. W. (1966). The pre-discharge ward. *Lancet; 2:* 1293–1297.

# Index